Managing Productivity in Occupational Therapy

D1358308

ΛΟΤΛ

The American Occupational Therapy Association

Rockville, Maryland

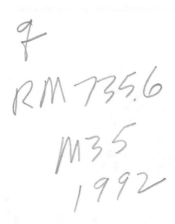
This publication is designed to provide accurate and authoritative information in regard to the subject matter covered. It is sold with the understanding that the publisher is not engaged in rendering legal, accounting, or other professional service. If legal advice or other expert assistance is required, the services of a competent professional person should be sought. *From a Declaration of Principles jointly adopted by a Committee of the American Bar Association and a Committee of Publishers.*

Printed in the United States of America

ISBN 0-910317-77-1

Director of Publications: Anne M. Rosenstein

Editor: Duncan Clark

Design: Robert Sacheli

Contents

Section 3: Productivity Data

Section 4

Contributors

Karen Chuck, MS, OTR

Assistant Occupational Therapy Manager, Alta Bates-Herrick Hospital, 3001 Colby Street, Berkeley, CA 94705

General hospital; Hand; Rehabilitation unit (outpatient)

Cathy Dolhi, OTR/L

Director, Occupational Therapy, Harmarville Rehabilitation Center, Inc., PO Box 11460, Guys Run Road, Pittsburgh, PA 15238-0460

Rehabilitation (inpatient and outpatient)

Tamera K. Humbert, OTR/L

Director, Occupational Therapy, Ephrata Community Hospital, 169 Martin Avenue, PO Box 1002, Ephrata, PA 17522

Mental health unit

Kathryn L. Kaufman, OTR/L

Chief, Rehabilitation Medicine, Psychiatric Occupational Therapy—Meyer 2-122, The Johns Hopkins Hospital, 600 North Wolfe Street, Baltimore, MD 21205

Day care; General hospital (outpatient); Mental health unit; Outpatient mental health

Mary C. Kolinski, MS OTR/L

Coordinator, Physical and Occupational Therapy, Northwestern Illinois Association, 521 Hamilton Street, Geneva, IL 60134

School system

Lisa A. Kurtz, MED, OTR/L

Director, Occupational Therapy, Children's Seashore House, 3405 Civic Center Boulevard, Philadelphia, PA 19104-4302

Pediatric; Rehabilitation unit

Ellen Loux, OTR

Occupational Therapy Director, Abbott-Northwestern Hospital/Sister Kenny Institute, 800 East 28th Street, Minneapolis, MN 55407

Cardiac unit; General hospital; Rehabilitation unit (outpatient)

Sheila Mack, MS, OTR

Director, Occupational Therapy, Henry Ford Hospital, 2799 West Grand Boulevard, Detroit, MI 48202-2689

General hospital; Mental health unit; Work hardening

Dianne McCarthy, MS, OTR/L
Director of Occupational Therapy
Deborah Lieberman, MHSA, OTR/L
Consultant
National Rehabilitation Hospital, 102 Irving Street, NW, Washington, DC 20010
Rehabilitation

Karen J. Miller, MOT, RMT, OTR/L
Consultant, 10709 Colonial Woods Way, Louisville, KY 40223
Private practice in mental health; Skilled nursing facility

Letty Sargant, MS, OTR/L
Director, Rehabilitation Service, Northwestern Memorial Hospital, 303 East Superior Street, Chicago, IL 60611
General hospital

Barbara A. Boyt Schell, MS, OTR/L, FAOTA
Private practice, 100 East Creek Bend, Athens, GA 30605

Sheryl K. Schwartz, OTR
Director of Occupational Therapy, Professional Rehabilitation Center, Inc., 12825 Flushing Meadows Drive, St. Louis, MO 63131
Geriatrics

Tina Scott, OTR/L
Occupational Therapy Consultant, South Carolina Department of Health and Environmental Control, Division of Home Health Services, 2600 Bull Street, Columbia, SC 29201
Home health

Beth Shea, OTR
Director of Occupational Therapy, Spaulding Rehabilitation Hospital, 125 Nashua Street, Boston, MA 02114
Rehabilitation (inpatient and outpatient)

Virginia Tully, OTR
Director of Therapies and Ancillary Services, Rehabilitation Hospital of the Pacific, 226 North Kuakini Street, Honolulu, HI 96817
Rehabilitation (inpatient/outpatient, work hardening, hand)

Kathleen Zahner, OTR/L
Supervisor, Occupational Therapy, Children's Memorial Hospital, 2300 Children's Plaza, Chicago, IL 60614
Pediatric

Acknowledgments

Many people contributed to this revision and we would like to thank them. First, Kathy Kannenberg and Truby LaGarde, National Office staff who served on the unofficial ad hoc committee and reviewed all of the materials for this book; the Special Interest Section Chairs, who offered their recommendations; the Publications Division at AOTA, which edited the manuscript and supervised production; and Wendy Schoen and Joyce Hynes, secretaries in the Practice Division, who did the real work of keeping us organized and on track. Finally, thanks to all the members who sent in materials for this book. We regret that we were not able to use everything submitted, but we thank everyone who supported this project.

Carol H. Gwin, OTR/L
Practice and Technology Program Manager
Practice Department

Ira T. Silvergleit, MA, MS
Director
Research and Information Department

Introduction

Carol H. Gwin, OTR/L
Practice and Technology Program Manager
Practice Department
American Occupational Therapy Association

In 1985 AOTA published *A Productivity Systems Guide for Occupational Therapy*. This was the first book on this topic to be offered by an allied health organization and was extremely well-received by the Association membership. It would have been easy to rest on our past success and ignore the urge to publish a revision.

Productivity data change frequently, and paradoxically they are often regarded in a negative manner. Who hasn't heard a colleague complain that the administration wants more service with fewer staff, and that money comes before quality of service? We in AOTA's Professional Services Department certainly had heard this in our telephone calls and meetings with colleagues. Nevertheless, we were also continuing to receive many questions about AOTA's productivity standards regarding the number of patients seen per day and for how many hours.

In addition, it was clear that occupational therapy services were being offered in new settings for which we had no objective productivity data. For example, were managers collecting data for the special units established in general hospitals since the advent of diagnosis related groups (DRGs)? Did outpatient settings have different productivity expectations than inpatient? What were the standards for rehabilitation, taking into consideration the "3-hour" rule of the Health Care Financing Administration (HCFA)? Were productivity expectations for certified occupational therapy assistants (COTAs) different than for registered occupational therapists (OTRs)? Were caseloads rising as our anecdotal information suggested?

Obviously, we did not have all the answers to the above questions, so the decision was made that the time was right to publish a revision. We approached our task systematically. First, two items on productivity were added to the *1990 AOTA Member Data Survey*. Second, we solicited assistance from the membership via letters to colleagues who were recommended by the special interest sections, contributors from our first book, and volunteers who responded to calls for help that appeared in *OT Week*. In addition, to minimize the problem of noncomparable information, a Productivity Questionnaire with a detailed letter of explanation was developed (refer to Appendix A) and sent to each contributor. Throughout, the intent was to keep the process simple and collect accurate information. Past experiences had taught us that productivity data were easily misrepresented.

To a large degree, we were successful, although admittedly, there are gaps in geographic representation and practice settings that were not overcome despite repeated attempts to rectify this. What did we learn? First, for at least general and psychiatric hospitals, productivity expectations as shown in the data have remained basically unchanged since the previous edition. Second, in contrast to 1985, the majority of contributors now consider documentation, travel, and family conferences as "billable time." Many of the contributors also include team meetings and preparation time. Third, everyone appears to be using productivity data in performance appraisals. Fourth, as in the previous book, many people may be using a modified AOTA Relative Value Unit (RVU) System for the purpose of billing, but most appear to be reporting productivity data in 15-minute units of time. Finally, we did obtain new data and were able to answer some of the COTA questions posed earlier.

Organization

This book is divided into four sections. It begins with an excellent chapter by Barbara Schell, MS, OTR/L, FAOTA entitled *Staff Justification Through Productivity Management*. This is the nitty gritty of productivity and will be especially helpful in assisting the new occupational therapy manager to get started in developing a system.

The second section contains productivity examples from our selected contributors. As you will see, they range from simple to complex. Some of the contributors go into a great deal of detail about their system, while others do not. Some have set productivity standards for all of their staff; some have not. As you review these standards, keep in mind that a "0" is interpreted as no direct service, and "N/A" generally means that there is no staff for these positions. In most cases, we could not use all of the materials submitted, so you may want to contact the contributors directly for clarification and additional information. This section is designed to give you examples of what your colleagues are using to obtain their productivity data and how these data are reflected in various management reports.

The third section contains the results of the 1990 *AOTA Member Data Survey*. For those of you being asked by your administrator how your department compares with other occupational therapy departments, this should help to answer those questions.

The final section of Appendices is really for loose ends. We have included the questionnaire used in compiling this book, a Recommended Readings section, and the Summary Report of the 1990 *AOTA Member Data Survey*, among other items.

I hope you find this book to be a useful resource on productivity. It probably will not supply all the answers, but it should serve as a good starting point, no matter what your area of practice.

Section 1:
Overview

Staff Justification Through Productivity Management

Barbara A. Boyt Schell, MS, OTR/L, FAOTA
Private Practice
100 East Creek Bend
Athens, GA 30605

In today's health care setting, change is the only constant. For the occupational therapy manager it is important to have useful information that can assist in determining the impact that changes in programs and services have on staffing needs. This chapter is intended to help the manager understand ways in which to collect, organize, and attach meaning to data about staff productivity. This information, combined with knowledge about relevant patient-client care standards, becomes the basis for determining and justifying current or new staffing levels.

Use of an effective productivity management system is important for all managers, regardless of area of practice. The materials in this chapter and throughout the book have been designed to reflect productivity approaches applicable to a wide variety of settings. As will be obvious upon review of the sample systems contained later in this book, individual facilities obtain and use information in ways unique to their setting. The reader can refer to the information in this chapter to understand the basic building blocks for a system that best meets the reader's own needs.

The Basics: Units of Measurement

In order to plan, it is frequently necessary to quantify various concepts for ease of communication. These concepts usually revolve around patient services received and approaches to quantifying personnel. Common quantitative concepts are described first for patient services and then for personnel.

Patient Services

Health care services may be organized by department as well as around specialties or programs. The data collected may be sorted accordingly. The division of programs or specialties is often determined by administrative decision. However, the occupational therapy department manager may decide to cluster services in ways that are useful internally (e.g., hand therapy, pediatric services, rehabilitation).

Units

A unit is a fixed duration of time that is spent in patient service. Lengths of units are defined by the department head or the setting.

Example: 1 unit = 15 minutes. One hour of service is 4 15-minute units.

Hours

An hour of patient service is often used when relating service to paid staff time. An hour of patient service reflects the amount of occupational therapy received by the patient, regardless of how much time it took the therapist to deliver the service.

Example 1: A therapist sees six patients individually for 1 hour each. That therapist generates 24 15-minute units a day in patient services or 6 hours of patient service.

> 4 units = 1 hour
> 24 units/4 = 6 hours

Example 2: A therapist conducts four group treatments a day, with 10 patients in each group. That therapist has generated 40 hours of patient service in that day.

> 1 hour group X 10 patients each = 10 hours patient service
> 4 groups @ 10 hrs/group = 40 hours patient service

Charges

Charges are the descriptors of service and the related billings that are generated when service is provided. The dollar amount of charges generated can be used as the unit of measurement.

Example 1: A therapist sees 6 patients individually for 1 hour each. The charge for 1 hour of treatment is $80. The therapist bills 6 hours, resulting in total charges for that day of $480.

> 6 hours X $80/hr = $480 billings a day.

Example 2: A therapist is responsible for four group treatments a day. There are 10 patients in each group, and each patient is charged $25 for group treatment. Charges for the day would be

> 1 group = 10 patients @ $25 each = $250/group
> 4 groups @ $250/group = $1,000 billings a day.

The kinds of charges generated can also be used as measures.

Example 3: Therapists might be expected to do one evaluation, two activities of daily living treatments, and four clinic treatments a day. These would be monitored by reviewing charge descriptors on billings generated.

Visits

A visit represents an occasion of service.

Example: If a patient is seen twice in 1 day, that patient would have received two visits.

Patients

A patient (or client, student, etc.) represents the number of individuals served in a given time frame.

Example 1: A therapist sees Mary, John, Pete, and Sally. She sees them each in the morning and again in the afternoon. She would record that she had 8 visits, but only 4 patients.

Example 2: A therapist keeps a roster of every patient she sees in April. She also notes, by date, each time she sees someone. She never sees any of her patients for more than one visit in a given day. At the end of the month, she finds that she saw a total of 15 different patients that month. By tabulating how many patients she saw for each date, and averaging, she finds that she averages 8 patients a day.

Personnel Measurements

Personnel measurements are used to reflect staffing by department, or program, or both. The following concepts are useful when budgeting staffing needs:

FTE

FTE is an abbreviation that stands for *full-time equivalent*. This term is used to represent the amount of time a full time employee works. A full-time employee is represented as one FTE, and part-time employees are represented as fractions of FTE.

Example: A person working half time would be .5 FTE.

Paid Hours

Paid hours are the hours for which individuals are paid, regardless of whether they were actually at work or on leave. Because employees, as part of their benefits, get paid for days when they are on vacation or sick, it is necessary to distinguish between hours paid versus hours worked (or productive hours).

Example: A full-time employee typically works 40 paid hours a week. A half-time employee would work 20 paid hours a week.

Productive Hours

Productive hours are the hours that staff members actually spend at work. They are determined by subtracting all paid leave (e.g., sick leave, vacation, education time off) that employees actually took from the amount of time that they were paid for work. To estimate, the manager can look at actual history in the department, or use amounts from leave policies and typical sick-time use.

Example: A full-time employee is normally scheduled to work 5 days a week for 8 hours a day. That person is paid for 40 hours. If he or she takes one day off for vacation, they would have only **32 productive hours**, out of **40 paid hours**.

In considering personnel measurements, the manager must be sensitive to all of these variables. With the current shortages of therapists, many managers are using part-time staff. This requires a method of equating staff efforts. Additionally, managers have to be aware of the differences between paid versus productive time. There is still a given volume of work to be done regardless of whether staff are on vacation or at a workshop, instead of on the job. The manager must be able to plan for coverage during these times.

The following two tables quantify common measures used by managers for budgeting.

Table 1.1 Paid hours for full- and part-time equivalents based on a 40-hour work week.

FTE	Paid hours/year
1	2,080
.5	1,040
.25	520

Table 1.2 Leave time (vacation, personal days, educational leave).

Weeks	Days	Hours
1 week	5 days	40 hours
2 weeks	10 days	80 hours
3 weeks	15 days	120 hours
2 weeks	20 days	160 hours

Average sick-leave use: 6 days/year per employee

Sick Leave (Short-Term Illness)

Most facilities do not expect employees to use sick leave except when the individual is ill. Therefore, in projecting sick leave, it is generally not necessary to assume that employees will use all of their allotted time per year (e.g., if employees are allowed 12 days a year, they generally will not be off 12 days due to illness in a given year). The author has found from experience and discussions with personnel managers that 6 days a year is typical usage unless employees are abusing sick leave by using it for other than illness.

Productivity

Productivity refers to the average amount of work generated by employees. It represents a relationship between the amount of time paid or worked, and any or several of the many methods of quantifying the services mentioned above. A productivity standard is a reflection of what management perceives as an average amount of services expected of a good employee when the employee is providing services of acceptable quality in an efficient manner. The occupational therapy manager should be very involved in negotiating productivity standards. Standards arbitrarily set by an administrator will not be effective if staff do not believe they are reasonable.

Developing Treatment Standards

It is apparent that productivity standards must be developed with a knowledge of treatment standards. Unfortunately, there are not ready-made treatment standards, as these will vary with the nature of the clients served, as well as the mission of the service-providing agency. However, managers can develop treatment standards relevant to their own facility by using the following resources:

Literature Reviews

Fortunately, more articles are being published that describe treatment approaches and correlate these with outcomes. This literature can be an important resource. The AOTA can often assist a manager in collecting these resources via its resource guides, which contain extensive bibliographies, and the on-line computer search option of **OT Source** through the American Occupational Therapy Foundation's Wilma West Library. University and facility librarians can help managers search the literature for relevant materials.

Consultation

There are many forms of consultation. One of the most readily available methods is to telephone colleagues who may have developed standards for their own facilities. One has to be sensitive to competitive issues, and, for that reason, one should consider calling facilities outside the immediate region. Many of the AOTA Special Interest Sections maintain resource networks with lists of individuals who feel they have expertise in specified areas. These can be accessed through the Practice Division at AOTA National Office. There is also a list of Professional Resources on **OT Source**, the on-line computer system. When extensive support is required, it may be most appropriate and well worth the expense to hire a consultant to come in and share his or her expertise. This can save the manager valuable time, help speed up the planning process, and serve as an educational tool for staff and administration alike.

Case Review

Another way managers can establish treatment standards is by review of typical cases. In reviewing cases, the manager can identify typical amounts of time required to perform evaluation, treatment interventions, and documentation and communications related to service provision. By looking for commonalities among cases that appeared to have satisfactory outcomes, treatment standards can be inferred. This approach works best when the persons involved have some experience with the kinds of patients or clients being served.

Once treatment standards are developed, they can be used to guide the identification of typical patterns of service. These then become the basis of planning staffing and productivity expectations. To illustrate this process, an example will be used, based on a rehabilitation unit's stroke program. (Further examples related to mental health and school systems are found at the end of the chapter. The basic system is applicable to any setting.)

Example: Stroke Program Treatment Standards

The manager of a hospital-based department was asked to assign staff directly to the stroke program, which was just being consolidated from the general rehabilitation unit. The department had been providing services to stroke patients for a long time, so she was able to use case review, along with information from other programs to look at patterns of care. Based on her analysis she generated the following descriptions of care routines in occupational therapy. Average length of stay is 4 weeks.

All patients receive:

1. Comprehensive evaluation, which requires 2 hours to complete (1 hour clinic assessments, 45 minute bedside ADL assessment, 15 minute documentation time).
2. Cognitive and/or sensorimotor retraining for at least 1 hour daily in the clinic (1 hour).
3. Weekly progress summary documentation (10 minutes).
4. Weekly staffing conference (15 minutes).

Additionally, the following services are also frequently provided, depending on the patient's needs.

1. Self-care retraining at bedside (75% of patients, typically seen 45 minutes, 3X/week for total of 8 sessions).
2. Homemaking retraining in ADL kitchen (25% of patients, typically for four 1-hour sessions during last week of stay).
3. Dysphagia program at noon meal (25% of patients, typically 1 hour daily for 10 sessions).
4. Feeding group (50% of patients at noon and evening meal for 45 minutes, 10 sessions).

Using this information, the manager can begin to construct a typical day or week for a therapist serving this population. By knowing the volume of patients, building in reasonable time for things such as patient travel, and accounting for one-to-one time versus overlapping or group treatments, the manager begins to create the expectations of a "good therapist providing services of acceptable quality in an efficient manner."

Productivity Expectations

Once the manager has developed a sense of treatment standards and patterns of care, it becomes a matter of using this information to develop productivity standards. When developing productivity standards for treatment staff, one generally has to consider three categories of time use:

1. **Direct time**: Time spent with patients or in chargeable service to patients (e.g., evaluation, treatment, splint fabrication).
2. **Indirect time**: Time spent on behalf of patients, but not in direct contact (e.g., documentation, reporting)
3. **Nonpatient time**: Time spent performing other job duties (e.g., ordering supplies, clinic maintenance, staff meetings, inservices, student supervision, research).

Direct time and indirect time can be estimated by using treatment standards and analysis of historical experience. Nonpatient time can best be assessed by looking at routine time demands on staff. It is not uncommon for an hour a day to fall into this category, with the time used flexibly, depending on the task at hand.

Estimating Productivity

As was mentioned earlier, there are a variety of units one can select to develop productivity standards. In the author's experience, the most common are 15-minute units and number of patients. In this section, we will continue with the stroke program example that was discussed earlier and use this data to establish productivity standards. We are going to assume that, at any given time, we have eight cerebrovascular accident (CVA) patients, with approximately two patients admitted and two discharged each week. From these treatment patterns, we can make assumptions for purposes of planning.

Example: Stroke Program Staffing Analysis

The manager had by now a good handle on treatment standards for this population and was ready to develop staffing requirements and related productivity expectations. She decided to analyze the patient care patterns as they would look for a typical week of services. She did this by laying out all the patients' weekly schedules for occupational therapy. She then developed the chart below, using the following categories:

- **Direct services**: A list of each of the service categories provided in a week. In parentheses, she noted the amount of billable time per patient (in 15- minute units), and the intensity of service provision (how many patients can be seen by the therapist at a time) in this service category.
- **Total number of patients**: The number of patients who would receive this category of treatment in a given week.
- **Patient time**: The total amount of service received by the patients in this category. This was the number of units per patient multiplied by the number of patients (e.g., 20 units clinic time per patient X 8 patients = 160 units patient time in the week).
- **Therapist's time**: The amount of therapist time it takes to deliver the service (i.e., the therapist's schedule). Because some services can be delivered to several patients at once, therapist time may be lower than patient time. If a therapist

sees a patient individually for 1 hour, it takes 1 hour of the therapist's time. If a therapist has a group of five patients, and this group lasts 1 hour, it still only takes 1 hour of therapist time (e.g., 20 units of clinic time at a 2:1 ratio only requires 10 units of therapist time per patient. 10 units X 8 patients = 80 units of therapist time per week).

For both patients and therapists, the time used is expressed in units, which equal 15 minutes. Later these units are converted to hours for ease of comparison to work hours. Additionally, the manager noted at the end of each service line whether the service could be done by an OTR only or by a combination of OTR/COTA personnel. This will help later in determining staffing levels.

Table 1.3 Analysis of direct time.

Direct services	Total number of patients	Units of patient time	Units of therapist time	OTR/COTA
Eval. (7 units, 1-1)	2	14	14	OTR
Clinic (20 units, 2-1)	8	160	80	OTR/COTA
ADL (9 units, 1-1)	6	54	54	OTR/COTA
Dysphagia (20 units, 2-1)	2	40	20	OTR
Feeding (30 units, group)	4	120	30	OTR/COTA
Homemaking (16 units, 1-1)	2	32	32	OTR/COTA
Total units/week	N/A	420 units	230 units	
Total hours/week		105 hrs.	57.5 hrs.	
Average hours/patient/week		13 hrs.	7.2 hrs.	

Based on this analysis, the manager could now see that, if patients are seen according to the treatment standards described earlier, each will receive an average of 420 units or 13 hours of occupational therapy service a week. It will take a little more than 7 hours of staff time per patient to deliver these 13 hours of care. The amount of staff time required is less than services received, because some services can be delivered simultaneously to more than one patient.

Now that she had figured out direct time required by the caseload, she turned her attention to estimating indirect time. Below is her analysis of indirect time, again using 15-minute increments.

Table 1.4 Analysis of indirect time.

Indirect services	Number of patients	Total time	OTR/COTA
Eval. documentation (2 units)	2	4	OTR
Progress notes (1 unit)	8	8	OTR/COTA
Staff conference (1 unit)	8	8	OTR
Total time required		20 units	
Hours (units/4)		5 hours	
Average/patient (hours/8)		.6 hours	

She now had a good estimate of the average amount of time it takes to service these eight patients in a given week, as shown in Table 1.5:

Table 1.5 Summary weekly time analysis.

	Patient time	Therapist time
Direct services	13	7.2
Indirect services	—	.6
Totals	13	7.8

For ease of calculation, she rounded the therapist time to 8 hours. She began to consider caseload sizes:

- 1 patient = 8 therapist hours
- 2 patients = 16 therapist hours
- 3 patients = 24 therapist hours
- 4 patients = 32 therapist hours
- 5 patients = 40 therapist hours
- 6 patients = 48 therapist hours
- 7 patients = 56 therapist hours
- 8 patients = 64 therapist hours

How many patients should a therapist expect to carry? Should the manager assign a caseload that takes up a full 40 hours a week? Not likely, if she wants the therapist to have any time at all to contribute to the general operations of the department. Using the earlier assumption of 1 hour a day to attend to all the other things that happen in a department (and to allow the therapist time to use the restroom!), the manager realized each therapist really only had available 35 hours a week for patient care. Based on her assumptions above, each therapist would be able to handle between 4 and 5 patients. Since the manager knew that "in real life" there were always some cancellations, as well as variations in the kinds of patients at any given time, she figured she would need to build in some flexibility. It was time to look at levels of personnel as well as staffing patterns.

Establishing Levels of Personnel

Occupational therapy managerial judgment is required to identify which services require which level of personnel. The manager needs to consider several key questions:

1. What is the lowest level of personnel that can effectively perform this service? Consider OTR versus COTA, novice practitioner versus experienced clinician, and special training required. Are there tasks that aides or volunteers can perform, freeing therapy staff to concentrate their expertise?

2. How frequent is the demand for this service, and does it follow predictable patterns? The answer to this question helps the manager decide whether to put a premium on flexibility. OTRs are generally the most flexible category of staff, because they can perform all levels of service (evaluation and treatment). They are, however, the most expensive resource. Therefore, if there are sufficient numbers of services that will only require treatment services within the scope of COTA practice, the manager should use more COTA personnel. For instance, if self-care retraining services (in which COTAs could help) is only a sporadic caseload in a facility, and the rest of services required are mostly evaluative in nature, it may be more cost-efficient to use an OTR who can provide any of the services. However, if there are several caseloads where treatment services can appropriately be delivered by a COTA, and the scheduling of these services can be managed to spread them throughout a work day, then it makes good sense to use a COTA.

3. What are the willingness and skill level of OTR staff to supervise COTAs and supportive staff? Effective use of various levels of personnel requires that individuals have the communication and basic supervisory abilities to use "extenders" of services effectively. Additionally, time for this supervision to occur must be factored into the estimates of productivity.

4. What is the realistic availability of COTAs? If they are not available and other supportive staff are used to extend services, issues such as licensure regulations, training, and liability must be considered.

The manager has an obligation, both to the organization and to society, to provide quality services at the lowest feasible cost. Conscientious attention to staffing levels and to various staffing options is critical to meeting this obligation.

Example: Stroke Program Personnel Levels

The manager had already determined that some aspects of the stroke treatment could be delivered by a COTA. By analyzing her data in a different way, she was able to estimate how much therapist time could possibly be either OTR or COTA time. She went back and highlighted those services in her charts and added up the number of hours, as shown in Table 1.6.

Table 1.6 OTR/COTA time analysis.

Direct services	Total number of patients	Units of patient time	Units of therapist time	OTR/COTA
Eval. (7 units, 1-1)	2	14	14	OTR
Clinic (20 units, 2-1)	**8**	**160**	**80**	**OTR/COTA**
ADL (9 units, 1-1)	**6**	**54**	**54**	**OTR/COTA**
Dysphagia (20 units, 2-1)	2	40	20	OTR
Feeding (30 units, group)	**4**	**120**	**30**	**OTR/COTA**
Homemaking (16 units, 1-1)	**2**	**32**	**32**	**OTR/COTA**
Total units/week	N/A	420 units	230 units	
Total hours/week		105 hrs.	57.5 hrs.	
Average hours/patient/week		13 hrs.	7.2 hrs.	

Indirect services	Number of patients	Total time	OTR/COTA
Eval. documentation (2units)	2	4	OTR
Progress notes (1unit)	**8**	**8**	**OTR/COTA**
Staff conference (1 unit)	8	8	OTR
Total time required		20 units	
Hours (units/4)		5 hours	
Average/patient (hours/8)		.6 hours	

She then summarized these, as shown in Table 1.7.

Table 1.7 Summary of OTR/COTA time.

Service	Units of OTR/COTA time
Clinic	80
ADL	54
Feeding	30
Homemaking	32
Progress notes	8
Total units	204
Total hours	51

Now she knew that up to 51 of the 64 hours a week required for this program could be delivered in part by a COTA. She knew that it was unlikely that all that time would in fact be the level of service appropriate to a COTA, because she knew there were portions of treatment that would require a knowledge of neurodevelopmental and cognitive concepts that were beyond the education of a COTA. Additionally, the OTR would probably be writing some of the progress notes, particularly on more complex patients.

Based on her analysis and her understanding of appropriate COTA roles, the manager decided it would work to team an OTR and a COTA together to manage the caseload of eight patients. This would have several advantages:

1. There would be adequate staffing to provide patient care, based on the expectation of an average of 64 therapist hours required per week, with 70 hours of patient-related time available between the OTR and the COTA.
2. There would be better use of salary dollars by staffing with an OTR/COTA team rather than with all OTRs.
3. It would be easier to cover patients when staff took leave, as only one member of the team would be granted leave at a time. In this way, the other member would be familiar with the patients.
4. There would be approximately 6 hours a week that could be used to help cover follow-up appointments of former inpatients, which would promote more continuity of care and allow the inpatient staff to see how their patients did on discharge.

Expressing the Productivity Standard

There are several ways the above scenario could be expressed as a productivity standard. If the manager felt that the scenario was pretty representative of typical patient demands, therapists' productivity might be simply expressed in this way:

> The OTR/COTA team is expected to carry an average of 8 inpatients. Each therapist is expected to treat 4-5 patients a day, providing services reflective of department standards for care of the stroke patient.

Because of the variation of patient needs, and the fluctuation in caseloads, it is frequently desirable to express the productivity standard in units or hours. This approach avoids arbitrary oversimplifications of care patterns (e.g., requiring all patients to be seen twice a day). Additionally, just expressing productivity by caseload does not give much information on how therapist time is actually spent. The use of standards reflecting treatment time assists the manager in determining if a therapist's load is running too high or too low. Examples might include the following:

- The OTR/COTA team is expected to average 14 hours of billed service per productive day.
- The OTR is expected to average 24 treatment units per day averaged over paid days.
- The OTR is expected to average 75% productivity (6 billed hours/8 hours worked).
- The COTA is expected to average 28 treatment units per productive day.

These are some examples of how productivity standards might be expressed. The reader will find many variations on the theme of relating patient service units to staff time.

Example: Productivity Standard for Stroke Caseload

Earlier analysis had shown that it took about 8 hours of therapist time to generate about 13 hours of patient services in a week. The manager divided to create a ratio and found that for every hour of therapist time spent, there would be 1.6 hours of patient service generated:

$$13 \text{ hours patient time}/8 \text{ hours therapist time} = 1.6$$

Since she had already determined that each therapist would have 35 hours available for patient care, she could expect that they would generate 56 hours in billed patient services per week:

$$35 \text{ therapist hours} \times 1.6 = 56 \text{ billed hours}$$

This was an average of 7 billed hours/day:

$$56 \text{ billed hours a week}/5 \text{ days} = 7 \text{ billed hours/day}$$

The OTR/COTA team would therefore be expected to generate 14 billed hours per productive day (that is, for the days they were actually at work). Because the team would share the whole caseload, the manager decided to express the productivity standard as an expectation for the team. It would be too cumbersome to sort out who did what on each day, and it was not felt to be necessary. The manager did tell the team members that she anticipated that generally the COTA would generate more treatment units, as more of the group and over-lapping treatments would likely be done by the COTA with this caseload.

Justifying Staff

As noted at the beginning of this chapter, health care today is in constant change. For the manager, that means constant reallocation of staffing and changes in staffing patterns. In order to ensure adequate staffing, the manager is frequently justifying staffing requests and decisions to administration. This process requires good knowledge of staff productivity, ability to articulate and support a rationale for treatment standards, and sensitivity to budgetary implications of requests. This section will address strategies that managers can use to maximize their likelihood of success.

Laying the Groundwork

The manager who has data available to explain current use of staff time has an important tool. By sharing with administrators the rationale for staffing assignments, productivity expectations, and variables affecting productivity, the manager demonstrates that he or she is able to effectively quantify personnel issues. Administrators are more likely to respond to requests from managers who consistently have well-organized data to support their positions.

Actions to consider include the following:

1. Collect productivity data routinely and summarize it on at least a monthly basis.
2. Analyze data by therapist, program, and department.
3. Develop billing descriptors to support your productivity measures (e.g., if you use 15-minute increments, use those in your billing as well).
4. Work with administration and/or the finance department to generate computer reports that relate to your productivity system. If this is not possible, get a microcomputer and train your secretary to use spreadsheets and data management systems to generate summary reports.
5. Notice trends such as increases and/or decreases in referrals or program changes and discuss these with administration early, so that time for planning is allowed.

Document Rationales

When requesting new or different staffing patterns, document your rationale fully. A good rationale includes reference to service patterns, expected productivity, levels of personnel, and benefits of staffing change.

Actions to consider include the following:

1. Ask your administrator what data are needed to assist in the decision-making process.
2. Document sources used to develop rationale for service patterns (survey of facilities, literature, case review, etc.).

3. Use charts and graphs to display treatment patterns and volumes. This helps administrators follow your logic about patient needs and staff time required to meet these needs.
4. Convert patient needs to staff hours, summarizing by expressing them as FTEs required.
5. Document options and describe benefits and drawbacks for each staffing alternative. There are generally several staffing patterns that will work, but some may fit department needs more effectively. Include such considerations as ease of hiring, turnover, availability of staff to supervise COTAs or aides, flexibility of pattern, total salary costs, and coverage considerations.

Be Realistic

It is hard to gain approval for additional positions when current positions are not even filled or productivity of existing staff is poor. It is also hard to convincingly demonstrate the need for permanent additional staff based on a short-term increase in service demands. These issues are further complicated by proposals that don't demonstrate sound financial thinking. For instance, if staffing is being requested to serve a population that traditionally has no insurance coverage, it will be hard to sell unless the manager also addresses alternative payment sources such as grants or charitable funding.

Actions to consider include the following:

1. Analyze and be prepared to discuss current staff productivity in order to demonstrate the need for more staff. If productivity is low, due not to performance problems but to the nature of the caseload, be prepared to discuss rationales for not abandoning that caseload in favor of one that uses staff more efficiently. There may be good reasons, but you will need to be able to spell them out. For example, a therapist may spend all day attending an outpatient clinic run by a physician and only generate 2 to 3 hours of billing for that day. However, if patients referred as a result of being seen briefly in the clinic result in significant volumes of outpatient treatment scheduled on other days, it may be important to keep the therapist in that clinic. Reasons to share with administration would include overall revenues as a result of patients referred and continued physician satisfaction resulting in increased use of hospital services by that physician.
2. Develop staffing requests based on actual experience in being able to recruit desired staff. If there are no COTAs in your area, and you have never been able to recruit one, hiring COTAs should not be your recommendation. However, document it as a possibility, and describe why it is not considered a feasible option.
3. Analyze the financial implications of staffing. This is done by looking at the following:

- full salary costs (salary plus fringe benefits)
- expected productivity
- expected dollars billed based on productivity
- expected reimbursement for dollars billed

By comparing full salary costs to actual anticipated reimbursement, you can see if this looks like a financial winner to your facility. The financial department in your facility should be able to help you estimate likely reimbursement for dollars billed. If you operate under a cost-based system, such as diagnosis related groups (DRGs) in acute care, you may need to analyze cost according the savings (i.e., quicker discharge), or because it will provide a service desired by key physicians who are important to the competitive edge of the hospital.

4. If possible, identify short-term options when it is unknown if demand for increased services is a trend or just an aberration for that period. Use of contract or relief personnel, summer help, and paying overtime to staff for increased responsibilities are all possibilities to consider. Determine from administration how long an increased volume needs to be sustained before it is considered a trend.

Use Good Timing

Be sensitive to what else is going on in your organization, and time your requests as much as possible to fit the natural flow of decision making. It is often tougher to gain approval for staff right after the budgeting process, unless some indication was made during the process that more staffing would be needed. It is also harder to get approval if an administrator is new to your service and hasn't had time to gain an understanding of department operations.

Actions to consider include the following:

1. Study the decision-making process of administration. Compare notes with other managers and directly ask administration for feedback and guidance on best timing options.
2. Orient all new "bosses" to your department as early as possible. Tell them about your productivity management system and ask them what information would be helpful for them to see on a regular basis to stay in touch with department trends. Try and meet with your direct superior at least monthly to discuss departmental issues and include review of productivity and service demands as a routine part of that meeting.

Two case examples have been developed to show how managers could analyze and justify occupational therapy staff.

Case study: New Gero-Psych Program

A new unit is being planned in which older individuals who have experienced a recent, significant decline in their functioning are referred for work-up and recommendations. There is anticipated an average census of 12 beds, with a typical length of stay (LOS) of 12 to 14 days. Most of these patients are insured by Medicare. The occupational therapy director has been asked to identify occupational therapy's role in service provision to these patients and to recommend staffing levels. She calls around to colleagues in the Mental Health Special Interest Section and the Gerontology Special Interest Section, and identifies likely services that are anticipated for these patients. She then has some discussions with the physician who will be the primary attending doctor and the nurse clinician who is likely to be involved. Based on all this input, she is able to estimate the following routine services:

- **Screening**: Brief interview and Allen Cognitive Level assessment of all patients.
  Time: 15 minutes patient contact
  5 minutes documentation
- **ADL Evaluation**: Intensive evaluation, with documented findings and recommendations for discharge planning.
  Time: 1 1/2 hours patient contact
  20 minutes documentation and recommendations
- **OT activity group**: Activities organized to meet clients' cognitive levels. Major purpose is to engage patients in purposeful activity and monitor their cognitive levels in order to evaluate success of medication changes. An average of 8 patients will attend the group.
  Time: 1 hour 6x/week patient contact
  30 minutes group preparation and documentation
- **Chair aerobics**: An exercise group held 6 days/week, co-led by nursing staff. The purpose of this group is general reconditioning of patients, with a secondary goal of monitoring gross motor skill and ability to follow directions for all 12 patients in this group. OT is responsible for 3 group per week.
  Time: 1 hour 3x/week patient contact
  30 minutes group preparation and documentation
- **Staffing conference**
  Time: 2 1/2 hours/week
- **Family conferences**
  Time: 3 hours/week

Using these data, the manager begins to make some projections about staffing needs. She develops estimates on services provided, as well as estimates of staff time to deliver that service. Note that these are not the same because of preparation/documentation time required, as well as the differing amount of staff time to perform individual as opposed to group services.

The manager decides to work with an average LOS of 14 days, and build initial data around how many hours it would take to service 12 patients for a 14-day LOS. She assumes that 24 patients will be served a month (since there are 12 beds and each patient stays 14 days).

First she looks at patient time. Each patient will receive an individual screening and ADL evaluation, and then go to an OT-run aerobic group 3 days a week, and an OT-run activity group 6 days a week. Since patients are not likely to be in groups on the day of admission or the day of discharge, the numbers in Table 1.8 have been adjusted:

Table 1.8 Estimated patient time/month.

Formula is: Patient time x Number of patients receiving service = Hours of patient service.

Patient services	Patient time	X	Number of patients receiving service	Hours of patient service
Screening	.25 hrs.		24	6
ADL evaluation	1.50 hrs.		24	36
Aerobic group	1.00 hrs.	6x/LOS	24	144
Activity group	1.00 hrs.	12x/LOS	16	192

Total hours of patient service received per month = 372

Now the manager needs to analyze this information to see how much staffing time will be required. This involves adding treatment preparation, documentation, communication time, and accounting for group versus individual treatment. To identify the indirect time associated with each service, she uses the estimates she obtained from her consultations with colleagues.

Table 1.9 Estimated staff time/service.

Patient services	Direct time	Indirect time	Total
Screening	.25 hrs.	.08 hrs.	.33 hrs.
ADL evaluation	1.50 hrs.	.33 hrs.	1.83 hrs.
Aerobic group	1.00 hrs./group	.50 hrs./group	1.50 hrs./group
Activity group	1.00 hrs./group	.50 hrs./group	1.50 hrs./group
Family meeting	—	.50 hrs./family	.50 hrs./family
Staffing	—	.25 hrs./pt./mtg.	.25 hrs./pt./mtg.

She then constructs a typical month's volume of services, as shown in Table 1.10.

Table 1.10 Estimated staff hours/month.

Patient services	Time/service	Number of services	Total therapist time
Screening	.33 hrs.	24	8 hrs.
ADL evaluation	1.83 hrs.	24	44 hrs.
Aerobic groups	1.50 hrs.	12	18 hrs.
Activity groups	1.50 hrs.	24	36 hrs.
Family meetings	.50 hrs.	24	12 hrs.
Staffings (.25 hrs./pt. x 12 pts.)	3.00 hrs.	4	12 hrs.

Total therapist time/month = 160 hrs.

Using the known of 2,080 work hours/FTE per year, and subtracting the estimated total leave time of 252 hours, the manager estimates the average productive hours per year to be 1828. She converts this to monthly productive hours:

Average productive hours/FTE/month = 1828/12 = 152

When compared with the estimate of 160 hours needed per month to staff the new program, the manager sees a difference of only 8 hours additional needed over 1 FTE/month. Since the two numbers are so close, the department manager asks for one FTE OTR to handle the program, as well as 96 hours (estimated 8 hours/month X 12 months) for use of float personnel or overtime to make up the additional staffing time that might be required. When the manager submits the proposal, the above descriptions of service, assumptions of volumes, and the various mathematical calculations used to arrive at the personnel request are included. In this way, administration can see this is a well-thought-out analysis, not just a guess.

Case Study: School System Contract in a Regional Medical Center

The OT director has been approached by a local school system administrator to see if the medical center's occupational therapy department could contract staffing to provide Occupational Therapy services to the local school system. The director is interested in exploring this, particularly because one of his pediatric therapists (who has had some school system experience in the past) has been on maternity leave and wants to come back on a part-time basis. The OT director consults with the AOTA National Office and obtains a copy of the *Guidelines for occupational therapy services in school systems (2nd ed.)* (AOTA, 1989). He also calls the occupational therapy curriculum director in his state, whom he knows to be a specialist in school-based services, to find out some of the particulars about staffing requirements for school-based services. These are some of his findings: Services can be provided based on the direct service, monitored program, or consultative models. These vary as follows:

- **Direct service**: Child would be seen for either two 30-minute sessions or one 45-minute session per week, with 30 minutes for a teacher conference. Because less travel time is required, the manager opts to build around the 45 minutes/child and 30 minutes/teacher scenario 1x/week/child. Where children have similar needs, they can be seen in small groups (i.e., gross motor) and meet with PE teacher 1x/week.
- **Monitored**: Services are provided under supervision of an OT. Initially, use 75 minutes/child to set up the program and train the service providers (i.e., teachers and/or aides) to deliver the program. Once the program is established (i.e., fine motor program), the OT monitors the program 30 minutes every other week.
- **Consultation**: The occupational therapist provides input to another professional for his or her own planning. Generally, it requires 2 to 3 hours/case to review the record, meet with teachers, observe the child in school activities, and present recommendations to the appropriate educational personnel for their program development and implementation.

Having a better understanding of the delivery systems in the school environment, the director calls the school administrator back and finds out the following information:

1. There are 10 cases awaiting occupational therapy intervention, based on the Individualized Education Plans (IEPs).
2. There is a total of $4,000 budgeted to cover the cost of occupational therapy personnel.
3. There are likely other children in the total population of 500 children who may need services, but they have not been specifically identified yet.
4. The school administrator would prefer not to pay for travel, but rather have it built into the rate.

The OT director then figures out an hourly charge for the therapist's time. At full-time, before going on maternity leave, his pediatric therapist was earning $35,000 per year, plus 20% additional for fringe benefits. He knows from talking to the personnel department that 20% is still an appropriate amount to use even for part-time personnel, as long as the individual works at least half-time. His pediatric therapist has indicated that she would like to work 2 to 3 days a week, for a maximum of 30 hours/week.

$$\begin{array}{r} \$35,000 \text{ annual salary} \\ + \$7,000 \text{ fringe benefits } (20\%) \\ \hline = \$42,000 \text{ full salary expense, full-time} \end{array}$$

$$\$42,000/2,080 = \$20.19 \text{ hourly salary expense}$$

From his networking, the director knows that $35 to $45 per hour is the typical rate charged for services to the school system, and after discussing it with his hospital administrator, he decides to plan on a rate of $40/hour, which will return an acceptable revenue to the hospital, since these are "full-pay" dollars.

Since the school administrator has a budget of $4,000, he can figure how many hours of service could be provided within the school's budget.

$$\$4,000/40 = 100 \text{ hours}$$

At 4 hours 1x/week (not counting travel time), services could be provided for 25 weeks, or for approximately two thirds of the school year. If a therapist spent 1/2 hour driving each way, this would be a 6-hour work day, 1 day a week. The department head thinks this might work well, because he could use his pediatric therapist to cover outpatient services the other 2 days of the week, thus giving him needed coverage there, where there is a waiting list. In making his proposal to the hospital administration, the manager includes the following information:

1. A summary of the request from the school system.
2. Description of availability of a staff person 3X/week.
3. A summary of the waiting list problem for outpatients and the lost billings that it represents, along with an estimated net revenue from those billings.
4. A brief mathematical calculation comparing the full cost of the new position with the projected revenue from the outpatient program expansion and the new program in the school system. These are then compared for the net revenue to the hospital.
5. A summary of benefits, which might include:
   a. net revenue
   b. retention of an experienced staff member
   c. potential increase in referrals based on visibility in the school system
   d. community goodwill from joint relationship between school and hospital.

Once the hospital administrator approves the addition of this part-time person, the manager will be able to present the proposal to the school administrator. The manager has kept the school administrator apprised of the general plan and knows the administrator will be happy to have someone for most of the school year, as there are no other occupational therapists in the area to meet the need.

Summary

Productivity management is one key to successfully staffing an occupational therapy service. The concepts presented in this chapter are intended to give managers some tools to use in managing staff and justifying the need for staff. It is important that productivity systems meet the unique needs of each department and that data are collected that are useful to management for quality control, productivity management, and the monitoring of trends important to management. Managers should resist the urge to collect data that are not likely to be used to meet an identified need. In this way they can avoid burdening staff with unnecessary paperwork. By incorporating productivity systems within available computerized resources, managers can obtain useful information with minimal staff burden and be prepared to respond to the changing environment. At the same time, they can help reduce staff stress by establishing clear guidelines on "when enough is enough!"

Acknowledgments

The author thanks Mary Brinson for her information contributing to the Gero-Psych Unit case study and Winnie Dunn for her information contributing to the Regional Medical Center School System Contract case study.

Reference

American Occupational Therapy Association. (1989). *Guidelines for occupational therapy services in school systems* (2nd ed.). Rockville, MD: Author.

Alta Bates-Herrick Hospital

3001 Colby Street
Berkeley, CA 94705

Karen Chuck, MS, OTR
Assistant Occupational Therapy Manager
(510) 540-1498

Type of setting:
General Hospital

Number of beds:
250

Total number of FTEs for this setting:
4

Productivity standard (in hours per day):
OTR Entry Level: 6.25 hrs.
OTR Inter. Level: 6.25 hrs.
OTR Adv. Level: 6.25 hrs.
COTA Entry Level: N/A
COTA Inter. Level: N/A
COTA Adv. Level: N/A
Manager/Director: 0 hrs.
Fieldwork Supervisor/Coordinator: N/A
Assistant Manager (Acute Site): 3.0 hrs.

Type of setting:
Rehabilitation Unit, Outpatient Rehabilitation, and Hand

Number of beds:
39 (Rehab. Unit)

Total number of FTEs for this setting:
6 (Rehab. Unity)
4 (Outpatient and Hand)

Productivity standard (in hours per day):
OTR Entry Level: 6.15 hrs.
OTR Inter. Level: 6.15 hrs.
OTR Adv. Level: 6.15 hrs.

Form A is the charge and progress note sheet. **Form B** is an example of a staff scheduling sheet. Form B identifies how productive a staff is, how much down time a staff has, and how much time the staff has to schedule a patient for the following treatment day. In an 8-hour day, the standard is 24.4 units (15-minute units). **Form C** is a worksheet used by the contributor. Expected workload (written in hours) is taken from new orders of the previous day. Expected staffing is taken from the expected workload by multiplying the expected workload by the variable standard of .3277. Actual workload is the actual amount of units of services made for the day. Earned staffing is obtained by multiplying the actual workload by .3277. Actual staffing is the actual amount of hours the staff worked, and the difference is obtained by subtracting earned from actual hours. This tells the staff if they are on target or have extra time for projects or meetings.

Finally, **Attachment A** is a sample annual productivity report. Note that in a 1-month period, each staff person has 5.5 hours of nonbillable time to be used for such things as inservices, staff meetings, rehabilitation meetings, etc. Although the staff uses a registry service on occasion, the goal is to avoid this because of the high costs.

All forms and attachments in this section are courtesy of Alta Bates-Herrick Hospital, Berkeley, CA. Reprinted with permission.

Continues on next page

COTA Entry Level: 5.0 hrs.
COTA Inter. Level: 5.0 hrs.
COTA Adv. Level: 5.5 hrs.
Manager/Director: 0 hrs.
Fieldwork Supervisor/Coordinator
(Rehab. Unit-Clinical Coordinator): 5.25 hrs.
Assistant Manager (Rehab. Unit): 3.0 hrs.

OCCUPATIONAL THERAPY

TRTMT # ☐ am / pm

IP		OP	
8109 ☐ VF EVAL—15 MIN		☐ 8150	
8110 ☐ ADL EVAL—15 MIN		☐ 8125	
8111 ☐ ADL EVAL—30 MIN		☐ 8126	
8112 ☐ ADL EVAL—EA ADD'L 15 MIN		☐ 8127	
8113 ☐ UE EVAL—15 MIN		☐ 8128	
8114 ☐ UE EVAL—30 MIN		☐ 8129	
8115 ☐ UE EVAL—EA ADD'L 15 MIN		☐ 8130	
8123 ☐ ADL TRNG—15 MIN		☐ 8138	
8124 ☐ TRNG—EA ADD'L 15 MIN		☐ 8139	
8116 ☐ THER EX—15 MIN		☐ 8131	
8117 ☐ NEURO RE–ED—15 MIN		☐ 8132	
8118 ☐ FUNC ACTIV—15 MIN		☐ 8133	
8119 ☐ GRMNT MEAS—30 MIN		☐ 8134	
8120 ☐ EA ADD'L 15 MIN		☐ 8135	
8278 ☐ SPLINTING—15 MIN		☐ 8277	
8101 ☐ ADL GRP—30 MIN		☐ 8142	
8102 ☐ ADL GRP EA ADD'L 15 MIN		☐ 8143	
8103 ☐ THER EX—15 MIN BU (1.2 UOS)		☐ 8144	
8104 ☐ GRMNT MEAS—30 MIN BU (2.2 UOS)		☐ 8145	
8105 ☐ EA ADD'L 15 MIN BU (1.2 UOS)		☐ 8146	
8106 ☐ EQUIPMENT & SUPPLIES		☐ 8147	
9091 ☐ WRITTEN REPORT 10 MIN		☐ 9096	
9089 ☐ CALL REPORT 5 MIN		☐ 9094	
9090 ☐ CASE CONFERENCE 15 MIN		☐ 9095	
9092 ☐ EDUCATIONAL SUPPLIES		☐ 9097	
☐ MISSED APPOINTMENTS		☐ 9098	
9093 ☐ UNIVERSAL PRECAUTIONS		☐ 9099	

SIGNATURE X   DATE OF SERVICE

EQUIPMENT   AMOUNT $ $

ACCOUNT NO.
NAME
RECORD NO.   BIRTHDATE
PHYSICIAN

ALTA BATES HOSPITAL   3001 COLBY ST., BERKELEY, CA 94705

OCCUPATIONAL THERAPY

TRTMT # ☐ am / pm

IP		OP	
8109 ☐ VF EVAL—15 MIN		☐ 8150	
8110 ☐ ADL EVAL—15 MIN		☐ 8125	
8111 ☐ ADL EVAL—30 MIN		☐ 8126	
8112 ☐ ADL EVAL—EA ADD'L 15 MIN		☐ 8127	
8113 ☐ UE EVAL—15 MIN		☐ 8128	
8114 ☐ UE EVAL—30 MIN		☐ 8129	
8115 ☐ UE EVAL—EA ADD'L 15 MIN		☐ 8130	
8123 ☐ ADL TRNG—15 MIN		☐ 8138	
8124 ☐ TRNG—EA ADD'L 15 MIN		☐ 8139	
8116 ☐ THER EX—15 MIN		☐ 8131	
8117 ☐ NEURO RE–ED—15 MIN		☐ 8132	
8118 ☐ FUNC ACTIV—15 MIN		☐ 8133	
8119 ☐ GRMNT MEAS—30 MIN		☐ 8134	
8120 ☐ EA ADD'L 15 MIN		☐ 8135	
8278 ☐ SPLINTING—15 MIN		☐ 8277	
8101 ☐ ADL GRP—30 MIN		☐ 8142	
8102 ☐ ADL GRP EA ADD'L 15 MIN		☐ 8143	
8103 ☐ THER EX—15 MIN BU (1.2 UOS)		☐ 8144	
8104 ☐ GRMNT MEAS—30 MIN BU (2.2 UOS)		☐ 8145	
8105 ☐ EA ADD'L 15 MIN BU (1.2 UOS)		☐ 8146	
8106 ☐ EQUIPMENT & SUPPLIES		☐ 8147	
9091 ☐ WRITTEN REPORT 10 MIN		☐ 9096	
9089 ☐ CALL REPORT 5 MIN		☐ 9094	
9090 ☐ CASE CONFERENCE 15 MIN		☐ 9095	
9092 ☐ EDUCATIONAL SUPPLIES		☐ 9097	
☐ MISSED APPOINTMENTS		☐ 9098	
9093 ☐ UNIVERSAL PRECAUTIONS		☐ 9099	

SIGNATURE X   DATE OF SERVICE

EQUIPMENT   AMOUNT $ $

ACCOUNT NO.
NAME
RECORD NO.   BIRTHDATE
PHYSICIAN

ALTA BATES HOSPITAL   3001 COLBY ST., BERKELEY, CA 94705

MEDICAL RECORDS

Form B

ABH REHABILITATION SERVICES MASTER RECORD

EXAMPLE

DATE: 3/15/91
ASSIGNED THERAPIST: Karen
HOURS: 7:30 – 4:00

MORNING

SCHED. TIME	PATIENT NAME	ROOM NO.	Tx	15 M UNIT ASGN	8:00	9:00	10:00	11:00	12:00	15 M UNIT CHRG	COMMENTS
8:00	Jones	4123	eval	3	XXXXC					3	
8:45	Smith	4106	ADL	3		X XX				2	
9:30	Gordon	4101	ther ex	3		XXXXXX				4	
10:15	James	4124	eval	3			XXXXX			4	
11:00	Sales	4103	ADL	3				XXXX		3	
11:45	Miles	6203	feed	3					TXX	2	
12:30	lunch										
				SUBTOTAL 18						SUBTOTAL 17	

AFTERNOON

SCHED. TIME	PATIENT NAME	ROOM NO.	Tx	15 M UNIT ASGN	12:30	1:00	2:00	3:00	4:00	5:00	15 M UNIT CHRG	COMMENTS
1:30	Scheduling											
1:45	Jones	4123	ADL	3			TXXXXX				3	
2:30	Mullen	6703	ther ex	3				R			0	0 Phoned office to get new pt
3:15	Mills	6402	ther	3				XXXX			3	
3:30	Samsone	6403	ADL						0 XX		2	
				TOTAL 9							TOTAL 8	

G:GONE DC:DISCHARGED R:REFUSED RN:RN PROCEDURE T:TRAVEL B:BATHROOM M:MEDICAL C:CONSULT P:PRIORITIZING O:OTHER

Service Line: O. T. Date: 6/17/91 – 6/29/91

Date	Expected Workload	Expected Staffing	Actual Workload	"Earned" Staffing	Actual Staffing	Difference
6/17	100	32.77	101.36	33.22	31	+2.22
6/18	140	45.9	136.52	44.06	45.25	-1.19
6/19	90	295	93.68	30.70	37.25	-6.55
6/20	95	31.1	95.74	31.37	30	-1.37
6/21	76	25	75.68	24.8	25.5	-.70
6/22	26	8.5	26.04	8.5	8.0	+.5
6/24	95	31.13	94.54	30.98	29.5	1.48
6/25	95	31.13	95.72	30.5	29.25	1.25
6/26	91	29.8	91.04	29.75	28.75	1.0
6/27	90	29.5	88.06	28.86	30.5	-1.64
6/28	75	24.6	77.02	25.24	11.5	13.74
6/29	22	72	22.68	7.43	7.5	-.07
						8.67

01/07/91
Cost Center: 17210 Occupational Therapy
Manager 1: K. Chuck
Manager 2: J. Grebe
Manager 3: C. Hirsch-Butler

Alta Bates - Herrick Hospital Productivity Management Report

(PMR)

Pay Period	Date Ending	Fixed Budget Hours Prod	N-Prod	Paid	Volume Budget	Actual	Standards Fixed Portion	Variable hrs/Unit	Earned Prod Hours	Agency & Registry Hours	Actual Hours Prod	N-Prod	Paid	Productive Performance Ratio	FTE Var Productive Efficiency	Volume	Bgt Adj	Total	N-Prod	Adjusted Paid	Adjusted Performance Ratio
1	01/13/90	525	120	645	1384	981	68.0	0.3307	392	51	394	48	442	99.5	-0.02	1.67	0.00	1.65	0.90	0.88	115.8
2	01/27/90	525	120	645	1384	954	68.0	0.3307	383	76	379	40	420	101.1	0.05	1.78	0.00	1.83	0.99	1.05	119.9
3	02/10/90	497	113	610	1298	865	68.0	0.3307	354	64	357	29	386	98.9	-0.05	1.79	-0.01	1.73	1.06	1.01	120.9
4	02/24/90	497	113	610	1298	748	68.0	0.3307	315	38	317	132	450	99.4	-0.02	2.27	-0.01	2.24	-0.24	-0.26	95.4
5	03/10/90	493	95	588	1286	1240	68.0	0.3307	478	139	461	12	474	103.5	0.21	0.19	0.00	0.40	1.04	1.24	120.9
6	03/24/90	493	95	588	1286	1157	68.0	0.3307	450	152	453	70	523	99.4	-0.03	0.53	0.00	0.50	0.32	0.29	104.4
7	04/07/90	461	111	572	1192	1048	68.0	0.3307	414	94	410	44	455	101.1	0.06	0.59	0.00	0.65	0.83	0.89	115.6
8	04/21/90	461	111	572	1192	780	68.0	0.3307	326	48	329	49	378	99.0	-0.04	1.70	0.00	1.66	0.78	0.74	115.6
9	05/05/90	444	102	547	1141	807	68.0	0.3307	335	66	338	57	396	99.0	-0.04	1.38	0.00	1.34	0.56	0.52	110.4
10	05/19/90	444	102	547	1141	853	68.0	0.3307	350	83	338	82	421	103.4	0.15	1.19	0.00	1.34	0.25	0.39	107.4
11	06/02/90	436	141	578	1116	717	68.0	0.3307	305	29	307	57	365	99.2	-0.03	1.65	-0.01	1.61	1.05	1.02	122.3
12	06/16/90	436	141	578	1116	690	68.0	0.3307	296	24	285	148	434	103.7	0.13	1.76	-0.01	1.88	-0.08	0.05	100.8
13	06/30/90	429	152	581	1093	896	68.0	0.3307	364	22	350	124	474	103.9	0.17	0.81	0.00	0.98	0.35	0.52	108.8
14	07/14/90	429	152	581	1093	779	68.0	0.3307	325	29	301	125	426	108.1	0.31	1.30	0.00	1.61	0.34	0.65	112.1
15	07/28/90	411	116	527	1039	805	68.0	0.3307	334	22	331	9	341	100.8	0.04	0.97	0.00	1.01	1.33	1.37	132.1
16	08/11/90	411	116	527	1039	854	68.0	0.3307	350	62	327	105	432	106.9	0.28	0.77	0.00	1.05	0.14	0.43	107.8
17	08/25/90	413	155	569	1046	775	68.0	0.3307	324	68	321	23	345	100.9	0.04	1.12	0.00	1.16	1.65	1.69	139.1
18	09/08/90	413	155	569	1046	759	68.0	0.3307	319	66	297	39	337	107.2	0.27	1.19	0.00	1.46	1.45	1.72	140.9
19	09/22/90	441	116	558	1131	843	68.0	0.3307	347	72	349	30	380	99.2	-0.03	1.19	-0.01	1.15	1.08	1.04	121.9
20	10/06/90	441	116	558	1131	780	68.0	0.3307	326	89	287	81	369	113.2	0.48	1.45	-0.01	1.92	0.43	0.91	119.7
21	10/20/90	435	123	558	1111	810	68.0	0.3307	336	71	270	105	376	124.1	0.82	1.24	0.00	2.06	0.22	1.04	122.0
22	11/03/90	435	123	558	1111	784	68.0	0.3307	327	76	312	70	382	104.9	0.19	1.35	0.00	1.54	0.65	0.84	117.6
23	11/17/90	448	131	579	1153	1025	68.0	0.3307	407	70	384	87	472	105.7	0.28	0.53	-0.01	0.80	0.54	0.82	113.9
24	12/01/90	448	131	579	1153	909	68.0	0.3307	368	29	297	141	439	123.8	0.89	1.01	-0.01	1.89	-0.13	0.75	113.6
25	12/15/90	470	136	606	1218	843	68.0	0.3307	346	69	313	99	412	110.6	0.42	1.55	-0.01	1.96	0.47	0.88	117.1
26	12/29/90	470	136	606	1218	672	68.0	0.3307	290	50	273	127	401	106.0	0.21	2.26	-0.01	2.46	0.11	0.32	106.3
Year-To-Date		11817	3232	15050	30422	22386	1768.0		9171	1671	8793	1946	10739	104.3	0.18	1.27	0.00	1.45	0.62	0.80	115.5

PERFORMANCE ANALYSIS		PERF RATIO	FTE EFFIC	REGISTRY HOURS	% REGISTRY	REGISTRY USE/UOS		SICK	VAC/HOL	NON-PRODUCTIVE HOURS INSV/ORNT	OTHER	TOTAL	%NON-PROD TO PAID HOURS
1990	THIS PAY PERIOD	106.0%	0.21	50	18.4%	0.0		0	118	9	0	127	31.8%
	YEAR-TO-DATE	104.2%	0.18	1671	19.0%	0.0		413	1164	189	179	1946	18.1%
1989	THIS PAY PERIOD	103.6%	0.16	0	0.0%	0.0		0	128	15	16	159	31.0%
	YEAR TO DATE	104.7%	0.18	604	7.8%	0.0		147	879	155	278	1460	15.9%
% CHANGE	THIS PAY PERIOD	2.3%	31.2%	****.*%	****.*%	****.*%		****.*%	-7.5%	-38.3%	-100.0%	-19.7%	2.3%
	YEAR-TO-DATE	-0.4%	0.0%	176.4%	141.2%	128.5%		180.1%	32.3%	22.1%	-35.7%	33.2%	13.3%

If you have questions regarding this report, please call Decision Support at extension 1849.

Harmarville Rehabilitation Center

P.O. Box 11460, Guys Run Road
Pittsburgh, PA 15238-0460

Cathy Dolhi, OTR/L
Director of Occupational Therapy
(412) 826-2738

Type of setting:
Inpatient Rehabilitation

Number of beds:
200

Total number of FTEs for this setting:
35.4

Productivity standard (in hours per day):
OTR Entry Level: 7.0 hrs.
OTR Inter. Level: 7.0 hrs.
OTR Adv. Level: 7.0 hrs.
Manager/Director: 0 hrs.
Fieldwork Supervisor/Coordinator: 4.0 hrs.
OTR Supervisor: 3.5 hrs.

Type of setting:
Outpatient Rehabilitation

Number of beds:
N/A

Total number of FTEs for this setting:
2.6

Productivity standard (in hours per day):
OTR Entry Level: 6.0 hrs.
OTR Inter. Level: 6.0 hrs.
OTR Adv. Level: 6.0 hrs.
COTA Entry Level: N/A
COTA Inter. Level: N/A
COTA Adv. Level: N/A
Manager/Director: 0 hrs.
Fieldwork Supervisor/Coordinator: N/A
Supervisor: 3.0 hrs.

H armarville's productivity system reflects the available days of time by OTR or OTR/COTA teams and the average number of billed hours of treatment per day. Note that COTAs are considered as a part of an OTR/COTA team. Each team member is expected to perform 5.5 hours of billable treatment per day (11 hours total). The productivity standard of 7 hours noted to the left is for an OTR working alone.

Form A is the therapist's record of the patient's attendance. It is a replica of the computer screen on which the therapist actually enters the patient's treatment charge and serves as the departmental hard copy. **Form B** is the individual therapist's productivity record, which is completed on a weekly basis. The therapist enters the total number of units billed for each day and calculates the totals at the end of the week. This form is then given to the unit supervisor who completes a summary report (**Form C**). Finally, **Attachment A** is an example of a productivity report format. The numbers in parentheses indicate the number of hours over (+) or under (-) the standard that the therapist or OTR/COTA team generated.

All forms and attachments in this section are courtesy of Harmarville Rehabilitation Center, Pittsburgh, PA. Reprinted with permission.

OCCUPATIONAL THERAPY DEPARTMENT
MONTHLY ATTENDANCE

Patient Name: _____ M.R. # _____

Month: _____ Therapist: _____ Code: _____

DATE	TXI	TXC	TXG	ADL	CEV	AEV	REV	HEV	SEV	DEV	FC	ORT	OT
1													
2													
3													
4													
5													
6													
7													
8													
9													
10													
11													
12													
13													
14													
15													
16													
17													
18													
19													
20													
21													
22													
23													
24													
25													
26													
27													
28													
29													
30													
31													

TXI = Treatment-Intensive   CEV = Comprehensive Evaluation   SEV = Site Visit
TXC = Treatment-Clinic   AEV = ADL Evaluation   DEV = Driving Readiness
TXG = Treatment-Group   REV = Re-Evaluation   FC = Functional Capacities
ADL = Bedside ADL   HEV = Home Assessment   ORT = Splinting/Orthotic Training

OCCUPATIONAL THERAPY

For Week Beginning_____

I. Record # of units billed per day and total/week

UNITS

Monday	
Tuesday	
Wednesday	
Thursday	
Friday	
TOTAL	

II. Divide TOTAL UNITS by 4 = _____ Total Billed Patient
Hours/Week

III. Record # of days worked this week

_____ OTR/L

_____ COTA/L

IV. Divide

$$\frac{\text{Total Billed Pt. Hrs./Week}}{\text{Total \# of Days Worked by Indiv. or Team}} \div _____ = \text{Billed Pt. Hrs./Day Per Indiv.}$$

_____ OTR/L

_____ COTA/L


```
Standard for OTR = 7 (IP)    6 (OP)
Standard for OTR/COTA Team = 11  (Average 5.5 hours per indiv.)
Standard for Supervisor = 3.5 (IP)    3 (OP)
```

7/89

Form 278/OT

OCCUPATIONAL THERAPY PRODUCTIVITY SUMMARY
FY_____ SIX MONTH SUMMARY
UNIT:_____

	THERAPIST NAME																			
	TX	DAY	TX	DAY	TX	DAY	TX	DAY	TX	DAY	TX	DAY	TX	DAY	TX	DAY	TX	DAY	TX	DAY
JANUARY																				
WEEK 1																				
WEEK 2																				
FEBRUARY																				
MARCH																				
APRIL																				
MAY																				
JUNE																				

Tx = Average # treatment hours/day for OTR or OTR/COTA Team

Day = Total # days worked by individuals (maximum 5 OTR, 10 Team)

OCCUPATIONAL THERAPY DEPARTMENT

MONTHLY PRODUCTIVITY

NAME	JULY	AUGUST	SEPTEMBER	OCTOBER	4 MO. AVE.
AREA 1 (BROWN)					
HIGGINBOTHAM	7.6 (+ .6)	8.6 (+1.6)	7.7 (+ .7)	9.6 (+2.6)	8.4 (+1.4)
KURTZ	9.6 (+2.6)	8.6 (+1.6)	LOA	LOA	9.1 (+2.1)2 Mo
WEINGLASS	8.9 (+1.9)	7.8 (+ .8)	9.8 (+2.8)	8.5 (+1.5)	8.8 (+1.8)
PHILLIPS(.6)/MERCER(.6)	7.4 (+ .4)	7.5 (+ .5)	10.6 (+3.6)	8.7 (+1.7)	8.6 (+1.6)
ELLIOTT	8.0 (+1.0)	6.2 (- .8)	7.1 (+ .1)	LOA	7.1 (+ .1)3 Mo
AREA 2 (SANCHEZ)					
SMITH	6.7 (+1.2)	7.7 (+2.2)	7.3 (+1.8)	8.4 (+2.9)	7.5 (+2.0)
FARMER/.3 FARMER	6.9 (+1.4)	8.2 (+2.7)	6.7 (+1.2)	7.4 (+1.9)	7.3 (+1.8)
ABERNATHY/.3 ABERNATHY	8.0 (+2.5)	7.0 (+1.5)	TERM	TERM	7.5 (+2.0)2 M
ZANER/.3 ZANER	8.5 (+3.0)	7.8 (+2.3)	7.5 (+2.0)	7.9 (+2.4)	7.9 (+2.4)
WOLENSKY	3.7 (-2.3)OP	6.4 (- .6) 2	8.2 (+1.2) 2	6.6 (- .4) 2	7.1 (+ .1) IP
AREA 3 & 5 (GREIDER)					
ROCKWELL	5.5 (=)	7.2 (+1.7)	5.1 (- .4)	7.1 (+1.6)	6.2 (+ .7)
KIRK	7.8 (+2.3)	7.5 (+2.0)	6.0 (+ .5)	7.8 (+2.3)	7.3 (+1.8)
BRONOWSKI	6.4 (- .6)	8.3 (+1.3)	7.1 (+ .1) 1	9.9 (+2.9) 1	7.9 (+ .9)
ATTLEE/JONES (.6)	5.8 (+2.3)	5.9 (+2.4)	5.4 (+1.9)	8.3 (+4.8)	6.4 (+2.9)
LINDBERGH	7.3 (+ .3)	7.0 (=)	7.1 (+ .1)	9.7 (+2.7)	7.8 (+ .8)
WILSON	7.9 (+ .9)	7.9 (+ .9)	7.1 (+ .1)	9.3 (+2.3)	8.1 (+1.1)
HULL/COLE	7.1 (+1.6)	7.2 (+1.7)	11.4 (+5.9)	11.5 (+6.0)	9.3 (+3.8)
AREA 4 (MADIGAN)					
O'BANION	5.3 (+1.8)	6.5 (+2.9)	6.1 (+2.6)	9.5 (+6.0)	6.9 (+3.4)
BURKE	5.7 (-1.3)	TERM	TERM	TERM	
NOLAN	6.9 (- .1)	7.7 (+ .7)	7.3 (+ .3)	9.2 (+2.2)	7.8 (+ .8)
KOPPERMAN	8.8 (+1.8)	9.7 (+2.7)	8.6 (+1.6)	10.7 (+3.7)	9.5 (+2.5)
FRENCH	8.6 (+3.1)	6.0 (+ .5)	6.8 (+1.3)	7.7 (+2.2)	7.3 (+1.8)

OCCUPATIONAL THERAPY DEPARTMENT
MONTHLY PRODUCTIVITY
Page 2

NAME	JULY	AUGUST	SEPTEMBER	OCTOBER	4 MO. AVE.
OUTPATIENTS/PAIN (BENSON)					
OSTROWSKI	2.8 (-3.2)	4.0 (-2.0)	3.5 (-2.5)	4.9 (-1.1)	3.8 (-2.2)
MILLER	3.0 (- .5)	4.5 (+1.0)	4.3 (+ .8)	4.3 (+ .8)	4.0 (+ .5)
SCHMIDT	3.1 (-2.9)	6.0 (=)	6.1 (+ .1)	5.4 (- .6)	5.2 (- .8)

Managing Productivity in Occupational Therapy

Ephrata Community Hospital

169 Martin Avenue
P.O. Box 1002
Ephrata, PA 17522-1002

Tamera K. Humbert, OTR/L
Director, Occupational Therapy
(717) 738-6474

Type of setting:
Acute Mental Health Unit in a General Hospital

Number of beds:
20

Total number of FTEs for this setting:
2

Productivity standard (in hours per week):
OTR Entry Level: 28 hrs.
OTR Inter. Level: 28-32 hrs.
OTR Adv. Level: 28-32 hrs.
COTA Entry Level: 28-32 hrs.
COTA Inter. Level: 32 hrs.
COTA Adv. Level: 32-36 hrs.
Manager/Director: 24 hrs.
Fieldwork Supervisor/Coordinator: N/A

This 134-bed general hospital has established productivity standards for both its inpatient and outpatient rehabilitation units and for its mental health unit. (However, for this publication, we have chosen to use only the latter.) All staff, including students, are responsible for completing the daily log (**Form A**) and the monthly tally (**Form B**) and submitting both forms to the director at the end of the month. All items on the front of Form A are considered direct patient care and all items on the back are indirect patient care and recorded in 15-minute units. **Forms C** and **D** are monthly reports that are returned to the staff.

The occupational therapy department does not bill for individual groups with services included in the per diem rate. However, it does bill for specialized evaluations. The RVU system used is modified from AOTA's system and is an indicator of possible stress load. For example, if there is a 90% productivity level in exercise groups, that would not be the same weight as a 90% productivity level in family conferences or evaluations.

All forms in this section are courtesy of Ephrata Community Hospital, Ephrata, PA. Reprinted with permission.

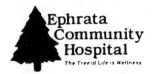

Ephrata Community Hospital
The Tree of Life is Wellness

Martin Avenue
Ephrata, PA 17522
(717) 733-0311

EPHRATA COMMUNITY HOSPIATAL
OCCUPATIONAL THERAPY DEPARTMENT
MENTAL HEALTH SECTION
PRODUCTIVITY REPORT - DAILY

DATE:													
INITIAL INTERVIEW/GROUP ASSIGNMENTS													
INITIAL NOTE, TREATMENT PLAN, COTE SCALE, HIS SCALE													
PROGRESS NOTE, TREATMENT PLAN REVISION, COTE SCALE REVISION													
DISCHARGE SUMMARY/DISCHARGE Q.A.													
FUNCTIONAL LIFE SKILLS EVALUATION													
O.T. EVALUATION (OTHER)													
FAMILY CONFERENCE													
BEHAVIOR MODIFICATION PROGRAM													
EXERCISE GROUP													
O.T. MEDIA I													
O.T. MEDIA II													
SKILLS GROUP/ADOLESCENT SKILLS GROUP													
LIFE ENHANCEMENT GROUP													
COMMUNICATIONS GROUP													
SELF-AWARENESS													
ASSERTIVENESS TRAINING													
BOWLING/RECREATION													
COMMUNITY MEETING													
EXPRESSIVE THERAPY													
STRESS MANAGEMNET													
RELAXATION TRAINING													
COMMUNITY ACTIVITY													
F.N.A.													
O.T. MEDIA 1:1													
WALKS													
CHAPEL													
PATIENT CHORES ASSIST													
BIOFEEDBACK													
TEAM MEETING													
TOTAL													

EPHRATA COMMUNITY HOSPITAL
OCCUPATIONAL THERAPY DEPARTMENT
MENTAL HEALTH SECTION
PRODUCTIVITY REPORT - DAILY

DATE:

ADMININISTRATIVE MEETINGS														
HOME HEALTH CARE MEETINGS														
PROGRAM DEVELOPMENT														
CONFERENCE/INSERVICE ATTENDANCE														
INSERVICE TRAINING														
STAFF ORIENTATION														
STAFF SUPERVISION														
QUALITY ASSURANCE														
RESEARCH														
PRODUCTIVITY REPORT														
O.T. DEPARTMENT MEETINGS														
BUDGET/EQUIPMENT ORDERING														
COMMUNITY-BASED MEETINGS														
TELEPHONE/GENERAL PAPERWORK														
DEPARTMENTAL MAINTENANCE														
LITERATURE REVIEW														
MARKETING														
SCREENING/INTERVIEWING PERSPECTIVE STAFF														
STAFFING GROUPS														
UNIT MEETINGS														
OTHER														
TOTAL														
HOURS WORKED														

1 UNIT = 15 MINUTES

Ephrata Community Hospital
Occupational Therapy Department
Mental Health Unit
Monthly Statistics

Month	# MHU Pts.	# Pts. OT Initial Eval.	# Specialized OT Evals.	Groups/Activities Lead-Co/Lead by OT	Groups/Activities Lead-Co/Lead by Students	Hours Biofeedback
July						
August						
September						
October						
November						
December						
January						
February						
March						
April						
May						
June						

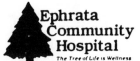

Ephrata Community Hospital
The Tree of Life is Wellness

Martin Avenue
Ephrata, PA 17522
_(717) 733-0311

EPHRATA COMMUNITY HOSPITAL
OCCUPATIONAL THERAPY DEPARTMENT
MENTAL HEALTH SECTION
PRODUCTIVITY REPORT - MONTHLY ANALYSIS

	RVU	UNITS	TOTAL RVU	MONTH TOTAL	MONTH TOTAL UNITS	MONTH TOTAL RVU
INITIAL INTERVIEW/GROUP ASSIGNMENTS	10	3	30			
INITIAL NOTE, TREATMENT PLAN, COTE SCALE, HIS SCALE	7	3	21			
PROGRESS NOTE, TREATMENT PLAN REVISION, COTE SCALE REVISION	6	2	12			
DISCHARGE SUMMARY/DISCHARGE Q.A.	6	1.5	9			
FUNCTUIONAL LIFE SKILLS EVALUATION	13	6	78			
O.T. EVALUATION (OTHER)	13	6	78			
FAMILY CONFERENCE	14	4	56			
BEHAVIOR MODIFICATION PROGRAM	7	2	14			
EXERCISE GROUP	5	2	10			
O.T. MEDIA I	8	5	40			
O.T. MEDIA II	7	6	42			
SKILLS GROUP/ADOLESCENT SKILLS GROUP	9	5	45			
LIFE ENHANCEMENT GROUP	9	5	45			
COMMUNICATIONS GROUP	12	3	36			
SELF-AWARENESS	10	4	40			
ASSERTIVENESS TRAINING	12	4	48			
BOWLING/RECREATION	5	6	30			
COMMUNITY MEETING	5	2	10			
EXPRESSIVE THERAPY	12	5	60			
STRESS MANAGEMENT	11	4	44			
RELAXATION TRAINING	10	4	40			
COMMUNITY ACTIVITY	8	4	32			
F.N.A.	6	4	24			
O.T. MEDIA 1:1	9	2	18			
WALKS	4	2	8			
CHAPEL	4	3	12			
PATIENT CHORES ASSIST	6	1	6			
BIOFEEDBACK	11	4	44			
TEAM MEETING	3	6	18			
TOTAL						

TOTAL HOURS WORKED   HOURS DIRECT PT. CARE
TOTAL MONTH RVU   ℅ HOURS DIRECT PT. CARE
                                            PRODUCTIVITY

ACTIVITY	TOTAL
ADMINISTRATIVE MEETINGS	
HOME HEALTH CARE MEETINGS	
PROGRAM DEVELOPMENT	
CONFERENCE/INSERVICE ATTENDANCE	
INSERVICE TRAINING	
STAFF ORIENTATION	
STAFF SUPERVISION	
QUALITY ASSURANCE	
RESEARCH	
PRODUCTIVITY REPORT	
O.T. DEPARTMENT MEETINGS	
BUDGET/EQUIPMENT ORDERING	
COMMUNITY-BASED MEETINGS	
TELEPHONE/GENERAL PAPERWORK	
DEPARTMENTAL MAINTENANCE	
LITERATURE REVIEW	
MARKETING	
SCREENING/INTERVIEWING PERSPECTIVE STAFF	
STAFFING GROUPS	
UNIT MEETINGS	
OTHER	
TOTAL	
HOURS WORKED	

1 UNIT = 15 MINUTES

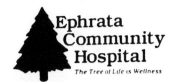

Ephrata Community Hospital
The Tree of Life is Wellness

Martin Avenue
Ephrata. PA 17522
(717) 733-0311

EPHRATA COMMUNITY HOSPITAL
OCCUPATIONAL THERAPY DEPARTMENT
MENTAL HEALTH SECTION
PRODUCTIVITY REPORT - MONTHLY SUMMARY

	TOTAL FTE	TOTAL HOURS WORKED	TOTAL HOURS DIRECT PT. CARE	TOTAL MONTH RVU	% TIME DIRECT PATIENT CARE	PRODUCT.	# ADMISSION
JULY							
AUGUST							
SEPTEMBER							
OCTOBER							
NOVEMBER							
DECEMBER							
JANUARY							
FEBRUARY							
MARCH							
APRIL							
MAY							
JUNE							
TOTAL							

The Johns Hopkins Hospital

Meyer 2-122
600 North Wolfe Street
Baltimore, MD 21205

Kathryn L. Kaufman, OTR/L
Director, Occupational Therapy
Department of Rehabilitation Medicine
(410) 955-6758

Type of setting:
Acute Mental Health, Day Care, and Outpatient

Number of beds:
146

Total number of FTEs for this setting:
22

Productivity standard (in hours per week):
OTR Entry Level: 18.0 hrs.
OTR Inter. Level: 20.0 hrs.
OTR Adv. Level: 18.0 hrs.
COTA Entry Level: 20.0 hrs.
COTA Inter. Level: 24.0 hrs.
COTA Adv. Level: 24.0 hrs.
Manager/Director: 0 hrs.
Fieldwork Supervisor/Coordinator: 18.0 hrs.

Productivity standard (in RVUs per month):
OTR Entry Level: 5700
OTR Inter. Level: 5900-6800
OTR Adv. Level: 5500
COTA Entry Level: 7000
COTA Inter. Level: 8800
COTA Adv. Level: 8000
Fieldwork Supervisor/Coordinator: 5500

Type of setting:
General Hospital and Outpatient

Number of beds:
900

Continues on next page

Maryland's productivity standards, measures, and billing are all based on the RVU system developed by AOTA in January 1979 (**Form A**). Daily billing logs are completed by the therapist for every patient seen as an inpatient or outpatient, with psychiatry using the same categories for individual treatments or evaluations as physical disabilities. Otherwise, patients are noted for the amount of time spent in various treatment groups (**Form B**), which have been assigned an RVU value.

All of this information is computerized, with the program automatically computing the RVU value, which is then multiplied by the cost per RVU to obtain the total cost of the treatment.

At the end of each month, a program is run to generate the monthly statistics. These include number of hours and RVUs for each therapist, each group (including names of therapists who led the group), each service (e.g., pediatrics, psychiatry, cardiac, etc.—inpatient versus outpatient), and a treatment record for each patient. In addition, there is a summary report that totals the RVUs, hours, and visits for inpatients and outpatients for each section (physical disabilities and psychiatry), and gives the department total as well. **Attachments A** through **E** are representative samples of these reports.

All forms and attachments in this section are courtesy of The Johns Hopkins Hospital, Department of Rehabilitation Medicine, Baltimore, MD. Reprinted with permission.

Total number of FTEs for this setting:
28

Productivity standard (in hours per day):
OTR Entry Level: 4.0 hrs.
OTR Inter. Level: 5.5 hrs.
OTR Adv. Level: 3.0 hrs.
COTA Entry Level: 5.0 hrs.
COTA Inter. Level: 6.0 hrs.
COTA Adv. Level: 5.0 hrs.
Manager/Director: 0 hrs.
Fieldwork Supervisor/Coordinator: 3.0 hrs.

Productivity standard (in RVUs per month):
OTR Entry Level: 5000
OTR Inter. Level: 5700
OTR Adv. Level: 3800
COTA Entry Level: 4700
COTA Inter. Level: 5500
COTA Adv. Level: 5100
Manager/Director: 0
Fieldwork Supervisor/Coordinator: 3800

MARYLAND OCCUPATIONAL THERAPY RELATIVE VALUES

Code Number	Occupational Therapy Service Category	RVU's per 15 minute time interval Patient-Therapist Ratio Categories		
		1 pt.	2-5 pts.	6 or more pts.
	I. Occupational Therapy Assessment			
001-03	A. Screening/Pt. Related Consultation	14	7.0	4.2
004-05	B. Evaluation	21	10.5	
006-07	1. Independent Living/Daily Living Skills & Performance	21	10.5	—
008-09	2. Sensorimotor Skill & Performance Components	21	10.5	—
010-11	3. Cognitive Skill & Performance Components	21	10.5	—
012-13	4. Psychosocial Skill & Performance Components	21	10.5	—
014-15	5. Therapeutic Adaptations/Orthotics	21	10.5	
016-17	6. Specialized Evaluation	21	10.5	—
018-19	C. Reassessment	18	9.0	—
	II. Occupational Therapy Treatment			
	A. Independent Living/Daily Living Skills & Performance			
020-22		16	8.0	4.8
023-25	1. Physical Daily Living Skills	16	8.0	4.8
026-28	2. Psychosocial/Emotional Daily Living Skills	16	8.0	4.8
029-31	3. Work	16	8.0	4.8
032-34	a. Homemaking	16	8.0	4.8
035-37	b. Child Care/Parenting	16	8.0	4.8
038-40	c. Employment Preparation	16	8.0	4.8
041-43	B. Sensorimotor Components	18	9.0	5.4
044-46	1. Neuromuscular	18	9.0	5.4
047-49	a. Reflex Integration	18	9.0	5.4
050-52	b. Range of Motion	18	9.0	5.4
053-55	c. Gross and Fine Coordination	18	9.0	5.4
056-58	d. Strength and Endurance	18	9.0	5.4
059-61	2. Sensory Integration	18	9.0	5.4
062-64	C. Cognitive Components	16	8.0	4.8
065-67	1. Orientation	16	8.0	4.8
068-70	2. Conceptualization/Comprehension	16	8.0	4.8
071-73	3. Cognitive Integration	16	8.0	4.8
074-76	D. Psychosocial Components	16	8.0	4.8
077-79	1. Self Management	16	8.0	4.8
080-82	2. Dyadic Interaction	16	8.0	4.8
083-85	3. Group Interaction	16	8.0	4.8
086-88	E. Orthotics	22	11.0	6.6
089-91	1. Fabrication	18	9.0	5.4
092	2. Material	Priced Manually		
093	3. Adjustment	12		
094-96	F. Prosthetics	16	8.0	4.8
097-99	G. Assistive/Adaptive Equipment	20	10.0	6.0
100-102	H. Prevention	14	7.0	4.2
103-105	III. Patient/Client Related Conferences	14	7.0	4.2
106-108	IV. Travel: Patient Treatment Related	10	5.0	3.0

(NOTE: Data recorded in minutes)

FLOOR: _____

GROUP: ASSERTIVE TRAINING

THERAPIST: JANE SMITH

MONTH: JANUARY 1991

NAME	PATCOM NUMBER	HISTORY NUMBER	THERAPISTS' INITIALS	NEW	M	T	W	TH	F	M	T	W	TH	F
						1	2	3	4					
MEYER 3														
Phillips, Tanya		123-45 67		1		60		60						
Franklin, Samuel		234-56-78				60		45						
Pratt, Lily		345-67-89				30								
MEYER 4														
Bolduc, John		567-89-01						60						
GROUP TOTALS						3		3						

PROGRAM NAME : RMMTH09

PAGE: 1

DATE PRINTED : 02/08/91

THE JOHNS HOPKINS HOSPITAL
REHAB MEDICINE THERAPISTS - HOURS AND RVUS SUMMARY
PSYCH OCCUPATIONAL THERAPISTS

Therapist	Hours	RVUs	Handwritten Hours	Handwritten RVUs	Handwritten Total
THERAPIST A	59.00	2898.80	45.25	2651.00	5,549.80
THERAPIST B	326.75	7168.20			
THERAPIST C	22.25	462.40			
THERAPIST D	0.00	0.00			
THERAPIST E	0.00	0.00			
THERAPIST F	26.25	948.80	62.25	3772.60	4,720.80
THERAPIST G	160.75	3653.40			
THERAPIST H	0.00	0.00			
THERAPIST I	321.75	6862.20			
THERAPIST J	29.25	691.20			
THERAPIST K	47.25	1593.20	43.00	2550.00	4,143.20
THERAPIST L	0.00	0.00			
THERAPIST M	163.00	5206.60			
THERAPIST N	32.25	874.60			
THERAPIST O	168.75	5259.60			
THERAPIST P	0.00	0.00			
THERAPIST Q	77.75	2222.00			
THERAPIST R	0.00	0.00			
THERAPIST S	49.50	1008.00			
THERAPIST T	0.00	0.00			
THERAPIST U	3.25	117.00			
THERAPIST V	159.25	4466.60			
THERAPIST W	273.50	6583.20	16.25	982.00	7,565.20
THERAPIST X	0.00	0.00			
THERAPIST Y	0.00	0.00			
THERAPIST Z	162.25	4170.00			

NOTE: Handwritten numbers represent data for therapists who work with both physical disabilities and psychiatry.

PROGRAM NAME : RMMTHO3

THE JOHNS HOPKINS HOSPITAL
REHAB MEDICINE THERAPIST VOLUME BY SERVICE
PSYCH OCCUPATIONAL THERAPY

THERAPIST	SERVICE		PATIENTS	ENCOUNTERS	HOURS	RVU
THERAPIST A	PSYCHIATRY	IN	24	37	26.25	1154.40
	PSYCHIATRY	OUT	7	7	7.00	134.40
	ONCOLOGY	IN	14	72	25.75	1610.00
		TOT	45	116	59.00	2898.80
THERAPIST B	PSYCHIATRY	IN	8	8	6.00	150.40
	PSYCHIATRY	OUT	41	432	320.75	7017.80
		TOT	49	440	326.75	7168.20
THERAPIST C	PSYCHIATRY	OUT	20	32	22.25	462.40
		TOT	20	32	22.25	462.40
THERAPIST D	CARDIAC SURGERY	IN	45	58	26.25	948.80
		TOT	45	58	26.25	948.80
THERAPIST E	PSYCHIATRY	IN	1	2	1.75	49.80
	PSYCHIATRY	OUT	51	153	159.00	3603.60
		TOT	52	155	160.75	3653.40
THERAPIST F	PSYCHIATRY	IN	2	2	1.00	84.00
	PSYCHIATRY	OUT	55	273	320.75	6778.20
		TOT	57	275	321.75	6862.20
THERAPIST G	PSYCHIATRY	OUT	19	20	29.25	691.20
		TOT	19	20	29.25	691.20
THERAPIST H	CARDIAC SURGERY	IN	48	104	47.25	1593.20
		TOT	48	104	47.25	1593.20
THERAPIST I	PSYCHIATRY	IN	67	206	163.00	5206.60
		TOT	67	206	163.00	5206.60
THERAPIST J	PSYCHIATRY	IN	20	41	32.25	874.60
		TOT	20	41	32.25	874.60
THERAPIST K	PSYCHIATRY	IN	28	203	168.75	5259.60
		TOT	28	203	168.75	5259.60
THERAPIST L	PSYCHIATRY	IN	39	90	77.75	2222.00

Managing Productivity in Occupational Therapy

DATE: 02/11/91

DEPARTMENT OF REHABILITATION MEDICINE
INPATIENT AND OUTPATIENT CLUSTER
PSYCH OCCUPATIONAL THERAPY

JAN 1991

CLUSTER	THERAPST	AGE GROUP	HOURS	RVU
SENIOR SUPPORT GROUP	▓▓▓	ADULT	6.25	150.40
	▓▓▓	ADULT	1.50	64.00
** CLUSTER TOTAL SENIOR SUPPORT GROUP			27.00	996.80
SOCIALIZATION GROUP	▓▓▓	ADULT	22.75	484.80
	▓▓▓	ADULT	13.75	264.00
	▓▓▓	ADULT	7.25	164.80
	▓▓▓	ADULT	3.00	96.00
	▓▓▓	ADULT	5.50	176.00
	▓▓▓	ADULT	10.50	336.00
	▓▓▓	ADULT	5.25	168.00
	▓▓▓	ADULT	30.00	576.00
** CLUSTER TOTAL SOCIALIZATION GROUP			98.00	2,265.60
STRESS MANAGEMENT	▓▓▓	ADULT	34.50	979.20
	▓▓▓	ADULT	17.00	412.80
** CLUSTER TOTAL STRESS MANAGEMENT			51.50	1,392.00
TOTAL			2,639.50	69,141.39

```
PAGE    1
PGM:  RHBVREVJ                                                                              DATE:  02/11/91

                         DEPARTMENT OF REHABILITATION MEDICINE
                            VOLUME REPORT BY REVENUE CENTER
                                     JAN 1991
                             FROM 910101 TO 910131
```

THERAPY TYPE	AREA	REVENUE CODE	PATIENT TYPE	PATIENT COUNTS	VISITS	TOTAL HOURS	MD-RVUS	C-RVUS
OCCUPATIONAL THERAPY								
(HSCRC CTR 7530) DAY HOSP	408	OUTPT	46	370	528.00	11,365.00	
* SUB-TOTAL DAY HOSP			46	370	528.00	11,365.00	
MEYER 2	443	INPT	255	977	1,216.25	37,761.60	
		OUTPT	96	605	895.25	20,014.80	
* SUB-TOTAL MEYER 2			351	1,582	2,111.50	57,776.39	
OSLER 1	416	INPT	333	883	782.25	47,827.00	
		OUTPT	115	275	274.25	19,469.90	
* SUB-TOTAL OSLER 1			448	1,158	1,056.50	67,296.90	
** TOTALS OCCUPATIONAL THERAPY			845	3,110	3,696.00	136,438.29	
PHYSICAL THERAPY								
(HSCRC CTR 7510) OSLER 1	442	INPT	758	2,661	1,811.00		18,869.95
		OUTPT	248	683	593.75		6,371.45
* SUB-TOTAL OSLER 1			1,006	3,344	2,404.75		25,241.39
** TOTALS PHYSICAL THERAPY			1,006	3,344	2,404.75		25,241.39

Meyer = Psychiatry
Osler = Physical Disabilities

DATE: 03/08/91

DEPARTMENT OF REHABILITATION MEDICINE
VOLUME REPORT BY FUNCTIONAL UNIT
FOR PEDIATRICS
YEAR TO DATE

FROM 900801 TO 910228

OCCUP THERAPY CC:714

THERAPY TYPE / SERVICE	PATIENT TYPE	PATIENT COUNTS	VISITS	TOTAL HOURS	MD-RVUS	C-RVUS
CHILD PSYCH	INPT	3	6	9.25	697.00	
* TOTAL FOR SERVICE CHILD PSYCH		3	6	9.25	697.00	
NEONATAL INTENSIVE C	INPT	24	202	154.00	8,954.00	
* TOTAL FOR SERVICE NEONATAL INTENSIVE C		24	202	154.00	8,954.00	
PED INTENSIVE CARE	INPT	27	116	108.25	6,486.00	
* TOTAL FOR SERVICE PED INTENSIVE CARE		27	116	108.25	6,486.00	
PED MEDICINE	INPT	86	438	392.50	23,711.35	
	OUTPT	12	19	25.25	1,564.00	
* TOTAL FOR SERVICE PED MEDICINE		98	457	417.75	25,275.35	
PED NEUROLOGY	INPT	66	255	242.25	14,763.00	
	OUTPT	5	5	4.75	339.00	
* TOTAL FOR SERVICE PED NEUROLOGY		71	260	247.00	15,102.00	
PED ONCOLOGY	INPT	9	34	34.75	2,160.00	
	OUTPT	3	11	8.00	519.00	
* TOTAL FOR SERVICE PED ONCOLOGY		12	45	42.75	2,679.00	
PED ORTHO	INPT	9	15	17.00	995.00	
	OUTPT	21	39	52.25	3,218.00	
* TOTAL FOR SERVICE PED ORTHO		30	54	69.25	4,213.00	
PED PLASTIC SURG	INPT	4	5	7.25	466.00	
	OUTPT	1	1	1.00	60.00	
* TOTAL FOR SERVICE PED PLASTIC SURG		5	6	8.25	526.00	
PED SURGERY	INPT	16	52	41.75	2,559.00	
* TOTAL FOR SERVICE PED SURGERY		16	52	41.75	2,559.00	
** TOTAL OCCUP THERAPY CC:714		286	1,198	1,098.25	66,491.35	

Northwestern Illinois Association

521 Hamilton Street
Geneva, IL 60134

Mary C. Kolinski, MS, OTR/L
Coordinator, Physical and Occupational Therapy
(708) 208-1049

Type of setting:
School System

Number of beds:
N/A

Total number of FTEs for setting:
35

Productivity standard (in hours per week):
OTR Entry Level: 24.0 hrs.
OTR Inter. Level: 24.0 hrs.
OTR Adv. Level: 19.0 hrs.
COTA Entry Level: 24.0 hrs.
COTA Inter. Level: 24.0 hrs.
COTA Adv. Level: N/A
Manager/Director: 0 hrs.
Fieldwork Supervisor/Coordinator: 0 hrs.
Educational Aide: 32.5 hrs.

T he Northwestern Illinois Association is a state regional special education cooperative that provides, among other services, occupational and physical therapy in approximately 250 schools over 10 counties. It also provides productivity information for 18 administrations.

For each student, therapists are responsible for maintaining **Form A** and completing **Form B** for students participating in the TAMES third party billing process. TAMES is an independent consulting firm that provides the third party billing system and manages claims. Therapists annually complete **Forms C** and **D**, which are used to determine staffing needs and activities for the subsequent school year. The coordinator completes **Form E** from data synthesized from the other forms to calculate full-time-equivalencies (FTEs) needed to provide services. **Attachment A** explains how to complete Form E.

With regard to the productivity standard shown to the left, note that one day each week (7.5 hours) is allowed for documentation, meetings, supervision, etc.

All forms and attachments in this section except Form B are courtesy of the Northwestern Illinois Association and Mary C. Kolinski. Reprinted with permission. Form B is courtesy of TAMES/HRS. Management, Inc. Reprinted with permission.

NORTHWESTERN ILLINOIS ASSOCIATION

THERAPY DIVISION

ATTENDANCE RECORD

	JAN	FEB	MAR	APRIL	MAY	JUNE	
1							
2							Student Name
3							
4							
5							
6							Program/District
7							
8							
9							School Year
10							
11							KEY
12							C = Clinic
13							CB = Community Based
14							EQ = Equipment
15							EV = Evaluation
16							H = Home Visit
17							O = Other
18							P = Paperwork
19							PC = Parental Contact
20							S = Staffing
21							SW = Swimming
22							T = Treatment
23							TC = Teacher Contact
24							TM = Team Meetings
25							1 unit of time = 15 minutes
26							
27							A = Student Absent
28							V = Vacation
29							CS = Cancelled by School
30							CT = Cancelled by Therapist
31							TA = Therapist Absent

SERVICE DESCRIPTION
PHYSICIAN/PRACTICIONER

TAMES

TAMES OF N.I.A.
521 Hamilton St.
Geneva, IL 60134

No. TAMES 33766

NAME					I.D. NO.	
PLACE OF SERVICE		TYPE OF SERVICE			ACTIVITY SERVICE NO.	

DIAGNOSTIC CODE: PRIMARY   SECONDARY

PROCEDURE NO.	TESTS	DATE OF SERVICE FROM	TO	TREATMENT SESSIONS	SERVICE DESCRIPTION

TAMES BILLING _____ _____
                Date   Physician/Practitioner Signature

COMPLETE ONE SHEET FOR EACH PROGRAM

THERAPY DIVISION

PRELIMINARY NEEDS ASSESSMENT DATA FORM PART I – 1990/91

RETURN TO DIVISION COORDINATOR BY _____

THERAPIST: _____   DISTRICT/COOP/AGENCY _____

SERVICE: _____ PT _____ OT   PROGRAM: _____

CURRENT FTE IN THE PROGRAM: _____

PROGRAM AND STUDENT INFORMATION

| SCHOOL/TYPE OF CLASSROOM | STUDENT'S NAMES IN PROGRAM/SCHOOL | BD | IEP'D SERVICE NEEDS | | | | ANT. TRANSFER | NEW |
			DIRECT WK/MO	CONS. WK/MO	MON. WK/MO	EQUIP/ADAPT. WK/MO/SEM		

NORTHWESTERN ILLINOIS ASSOCIATION

THERAPY DIVISION

DATA FORM - PART II

1990-91 NEEDS ASSESSMENT

THERAPIST NAME: _____

SERVICE: _____ PT _____ OT

Complete the following information to the best of your ability. Refer to your weekly schedule when applicable.

Indicate on the grid below, information requested in 1, 2 and 3.

1. Travel time PER WEEK for each assignment. Provide the number of hours of <u>travel only</u>, excluding therapy set-up and clean up. Travel hours are those hours traveled between schools and agencies. **DO NOT INCLUDE TIME TRAVELED TO AND FROM WORK.**

2. Total number of itinerant changes made in a week.

3. The number of schools you work in.

GRID

Program	Number of Travel Hours	Number of Itinerant Changes Weekly	Number of Schools Worked In

		Number	Program
4.	Number of students expected to be seen in clinics, (DSCC, MD), and the program in which the student is enrolled. (Refer to Program Guide.	_____	_____
		_____	_____
		_____	_____
		_____	_____

	Number	Program

5.   Number of diagnostics <u>completed</u> this year, including carryovers from 1989/90, in each assignment. "Completed" means that all diagnostic activities, including staffing, have been done.

	Hours	Program

6.   Number of hours per month <u>required</u> for <u>routine</u> team meetings, in each assignment.

	Hours	Program

7.   Number of anticipated hours per month for <u>required non-routine meetings</u>, including transitional planning activities, staffings, building meetings, etc. Specify purpose of these meetings below.

	Hours	Program

8.   Estimated parent consultation hours needed per month, done in addition to scheduled IEP'd treatment time.

	Hours	Program

9.   Estimated teacher consultation hours needed per month, done in addition to scheduled IEP'd treatment time.

	Consults	Program

10. Estimated number of written
consultation programs required
by this program annually.

11. Estimated number of written
programs needed for direct
service student.

12. State any recommendations which you may have for your specific
program(s).

Mary C. Kolinski, M.S., OTR/L
12/90

BE SURE YOUR NAME IS ON THE FORM

NORTHWESTERN ILLINOIS ASSOCIATION

THERAPY DIVISION

PRELIMINARY NEEDS ASSESSMENT FACT FORM - 1990-91

(Check)   PT _____   OT _____   PROGRAM _____

FY 90   FTE _____   DISTRICT/COOP _____

I.   DIAGNOSTIC ACTIVITIES   **HOURS REQUIRED**

     FY 91 _____ diagnostics
     estimated.

                          SUBTOTAL   _____
                                          Days

II   TREATMENT ACTIVITIES

     A.   Treatment time including student
          specific equipment adaptation
          and maintenance.

          DIRECT   _____

          CONSULTATIVE   _____

          MONITOR   _____

          NEW   _____

B.   Therapy set-up and clean up   _____

C.   Travel between programs   _____

D.   Medical/clinical consultation   _____
     (RDI, DSCC, MED, Etc.)

E.   Teacher/program consultation
     done outside of treatment   _____

                              SUBTOTAL   _____
                                              Days

III. TREATMENT DOCUMENTATION DATA

A.   Consultative instructional
     programs   _____

B.   Attendance/progress data   _____

C.   Reports/correspondence
     Annual Review Reports   _____

      D.   Other Correspondence   _____

                      SUBTOTAL   _____
                                                       Days

IV.   ADDITIONAL TREATMENT RELATED ACTIVITIES

      A.   School Meetings

           1.   Annual reviews   _____

           2.   Team meetings   _____

           3.   Other staffings   _____

      B.   Supervisory/other administrative   _____

      C.   Schedules/calendars   _____

      D.   Program/professional development
             activities   _____

E.   Parent consultation done outside
of treatment   _____

F.   Therapy equipment-general
ordering and maintenance   _____

G.   Treatment planning   _____

H.   Insurance billing   _____

SUBTOTAL   _____
                                   Days

GRAND TOTAL DAYS PROJECTED
FOR ACTIVITIES   _____

CURRENT FTE FY 90   _____

SUGGESTED FTE FY 91   _____

Mary C. Kolinski, M.S., OTR/L

crc
ndsasm.fac

NORTHWESTERN ILLINOIS ASSOCIATION

THERAPY DIVISION

INSTRUCTIONS TO COMPLETE

NEEDS ASSESSMENT FACT FORM *

1991-92 NEEDS ASSESSMENT

Complete each section of the Fact Form according to the instructions provided below.

GENERAL INSTRUCTIONS:

1. Complete a form for each staff member's assignment in each program.

2. Provide service information at the top of the page.

3. Calculate grand total recommendations for each program by adding all data for each service from split assignments (e.g. data from two PT's at Gates) and transfer onto the form, Occupational and Physical Therapy Services Projections.

4. Refer to the Needs Assessment Therapy Programs Guide attached, for names of programs.

I. ## DIAGNOSTIC ACTIVITIES:

1. Estimate the number of diagnostics completed by the therapist in each assignment, based on the actual number completed the previous year. You will receive this information from the diagnostic secretary. Information regarding diagnostics received from therapists functions as a cross check to determine whether significant increases in referrals are occurring.

2. Using the estimated number in #1, provide 7.5 hours per diagnostic (includes referral review, student classroom observation, physical performance evaluation, standardized tests, communication with team members, scoring tests, writing report and goals and objectives, and report-back staffing.

3. Subtotal days for the above activities. Enter next to SUBTOTAL.

II. TREATMENT ACTIVITIES:

Base calculations in this category upon:

* A 6 or 6.5 hour treatment day depending on the program.
* 144 days in scheduled treatment for a full time equivalency.
* A 9 month or 36 week school year.
* The current FTE.

(NOTE: use an average on direct service ranges and the high end on other models.)

A. TREATMENT TIME (DAYS)

Complete data from the Data Forms received from therapists. In addition to the specified information behind "New", add 45 minutes per week x 55% or more (depending on program history) of estimated FY 91 diagnostics to DIRECT treatment. Convert minutes to hours.

One formula which can be used follows in the EXAMPLE below.

EXAMPLE: Six (6) children are expected to receive 30 minutes of service weekly. Therefore, 6 x 30 = 180 minutes/week x 36 weeks = 6480 minutes per year ÷ 60 minutes per hour = 108 hours.

B. TREATMENT SET-UP AND CLEANUP

1. Calculate 20 minutes per day for a self-contained program x days in treatment.

2. Calculate 15 minutes for each itinerant change.

C. TRAVEL

Calculate number of minutes per week (on Data Form II) x 36 weeks ÷ 60.

D. MEDICAL CLINICAL CONSULTATION

Calculate number of clinical visits anticipated (See Data Form Part II) x 2 hours per visit.

E. TEACHER CONSULTATION (outside of IEP'd treatment)

Calculate 2 hours per week x 36 weeks.

III. TREATMENT DOCUMENTATION DATA

Calculations are based on a 7.5 hour day.

A. CONSULTATIVE INSTRUCTIONAL PROGRAMS

Calculate 2 hours per written program x 50% of the estimated caseload. Consider each program requirement to decrease or increase number, if necessary.

B. ATTENDANCE/PROGRESS DATA

Calculate 20 minutes per day or 60 days per year for a full-time position.

C. REPORTS/CORRESPONDENCE

Annual Review Report - Calculate 5 hours per report x number of total students. (This includes goals/objectives).

D. OTHER CORRESPONDENCE

Calculate 3.75 hours per month. 33.75 hours for a full time person.

Subtotal days for the above activities. ENTER NEXT TO SUBTOTAL.

IV. ADDITIONAL TREATMENT-RELATED ACTIVITIES:

Calculations are based on a 7.5 hour day.

A. SCHOOL MEETINGS

1. Annual reviews - Calculate 30 minutes for each review per student.

2. Team meetings - cite program - specific information, referring to Data Forms.

3. Other - cite program specific information.

B. SUPERVISORY/OTHER ADMINISTRATIVE CONTACTS

Calculate 18.75 hours for a full-time position (2 hours/month).

C. SCHEDULES/CALENDARS

Add 9.5 hours per year for a full-time position (3 hours initial x 1/2 hour/month).

D. PROGRAM/PROFESSIONAL DEVELOPMENT ACTIVITIES

Include 15 hours per year for each person.

E. __PARENT CONSULTATION (outside of treatment)__

Calculate 3 hours per month or 27 hours per year for a full-time position.

F. __THERAPY EQUIPMENT__ (general ordering and maintenance)

Calculate 27 hours a year a full-time position.

G. __TREATMENT PLANNING__

Calculate 30 minutes for each treatment day.

H. __INSURANCE BILLING:__

Calculate 18 hours per year for a full time person who is completing service tickets (MVSEC, District 300). Subtotal days for the above activities. Enter next to SUBTOTAL.

V. __GRAND TOTAL:__

Add the subtotals to determine Grand Total Days Projected for Activities. Divide by 185 to achieve the suggested FTE. Enter the current FTE.

* Data derived from in-house studies.

Mary C. Kolinski, M.S., OTR/L
crc
12/90
NDSASM.INS

Children's Seashore House

3405 Civic Center Boulevard
Philadelphia, PA 19104-4302

Lisa A. Kurtz, MEd, OTR/L
Director, Occupational Therapy
(215) 895-3785

Type of setting:
Pediatric Hospital and affiliated Pediatric Rehabilitation Hospital

Number of beds:
372 (72 Rehab.)

Total number of FTEs for this setting:
13.4 (9.5 Rehab.)

Productivity standard (in hours per day):
OTR Entry Level: 4.5 hrs.
OTR Inter. Level: 4.5 hrs.
OTR Adv. Level: 4.5 hrs.
COTA Entry Level: 5.25 hrs.
COTA Inter. Level: 5.25 hrs.
COTA Adv. Level: 5.25 hrs.
Manager/Director: 0 hrs.
Fieldwork Supervisor/Coordinator: N/A
Occupational Therapy Supervisor: 2.25 hrs.

T his pediatric rehabilitation hospital bills in 30-minute units of time and by procedures. To do their weekly productivity report (**Form A**), the therapists fill out the Productivity Monitor Sheet (**Form B**). The Productivity (x) on Form B is then plugged into column TDCH on **Form C** to determine whether or not the therapist has met the productivity standard.

Attachments A and **B** are examples of time/cost analyses done to see how much time was involved in doing evaluations (including preparation, scoring, documentation, etc.). Results were used as part of a proposal to increase fees for the evaluations.

All forms and attachments in this section are courtesy of Children's Seashore House, Philadelphia, PA. Reprinted with permission.

THE CHILDREN'S SEASHORE HOUSE

Department of Occupational Therapy

Departmental Productivity Monitor

Week Beginning: _1/28/91_

	CHOP	CSH IP	CSH OP
Monday	8.75	19.25	2.5
Tuesday	9.0	18.25	2.5
Wednesday	13.25	22.5	4
Thursday	10.75	21.25	.5
Friday	11.25	27	3.75
Saturday	1.75	5.75	—
Sunday	—	—	—
Total DCH	54.75	114	13.25
Minimum Expected DCH	58	110	9

revised 3/91

This data is calculated by a clerk, recorded from the charge slips handed in by staff.

CHOP = Children's Hospital of Philadelphia

THE CHILDREN'S SEASHORE HOUSE

Department of Occupational Therapy

Productivity Monitor Sheet

Therapist Name: _Staff therapist (example)_

ADCH Expectation (Average Direct Care hours/day): _4.5_

Month/Year: _January 1991_

Instructions: For each day, indicate the total number of hours billed for therapy under your name. (Direct Care Hours = DCH) Include charges submitted by students if charged under your clinician code number. Use NA to indicate any day that you were **not** present at work (vacation, sick, etc.). Form must be submitted to O.T. supervisor at end of month along with other QA forms.

			7		14		21		28
Monday		5.0		NA		4.5		4.0	
	1		8		15		22		29
Tuesday	NA	5.25		4.75		4.5		4.5	
	2		9		16		23		30
Wednesday	4.25	3.75		5.0		4.0		4.75	
	3		10		17		24		31
Thursday	4.0	4.5		6.0		5.0		5.0	
	4		11		18		25		
Friday	5.0	4.25		4.5		5.25			

Total expected DCH: _21 x 4.5 = 94.5_
(days worked times ADCH expectation)

Actual DCH: _97.75_
(Total hours worked during the month)

Productivity (X): _4.65_
(X = ADCH expectation X Actual DCH)
        TOTAL EXPECTED DCH

ADCH = Average Direct Care Hours

Revised 3/91

THE CHILDREN'S SEASHORE HOUSE
Department of Occupational Therapy

Monthly Productivity Report   Month/Year _____
(Monday - Friday)

THERAPIST	OT/ADCH EXPECTATION	TDCH	# DAYS WORKED	= ADCH	+/-

therapists failed to meet productivity standard _____

therapists exceeding productivity standard _____

THE CHILDREN'S SEASHORE HOUSE

Occupational Therapy Department

Time Utilization Study for Evaluations

Patient Name: _____

Therapist Name: _____

Evaluation type (check one)

_____ screening/consultation (15-30 minutes direct time with child)
_____ evaluation (involves formal assessment including the use of standardized measures)
_____ SIPT

Instructions: Using the following grid, place one hash mark (1) for each 15 minutes of activity. Activity does not need to take place on the actual day of the evaluation; eg: telephone call to school therapist to follow up on CP Clinic visit.

Intake: referral call, review of records, parent interview, etc.	
Direct Care: actual time spent in direct care/assessment of child.	
Scoring/Interpretation: scoring of standardized tests.	
Report: time spent writing evaluation report or preparing other documentation.	
Meetings/Conferences: team meetings to discuss results, parent conference	
Follow-Up: follow-up calls to referrer, parent, resource agencies, etc.	

Total time: _____

<u>Evaluation Time Analysis</u>

<u>O.T. Fee Revision</u>

	OT Screening	OT Evaluation	SIPT
# cases reviewed	9	5	3
<u>Intake</u>			
range	1/4 - 1/2 hrs.	0 - 1 hr.	1/2 - 1 hr.
average	1/4 hr.	1/2 hr.	3/4 hr.
<u>Direct Care</u>			
range	1/4 - 1 hour	1/2 - 2 hrs.	2½ - 3¼ hrs.
average	1/2 hr.	1 1/3 hrs.	2 3/4 hrs.
<u>Scoring/Interpretation</u>			
range	0	0 - 3/4 hr.	3/4 - 1 1/4 hrs.
average	0	1/3 hrs.	1 hr.
<u>Report Writing</u>			
range	0 - 1/2 hr.	1/4 - 3/4 hr.	3/4 hr.
average	1/3 hrs.	1/2 hr.	3/4 hr.
<u>Meetings/Conference</u>			
range	0 - 1/4 hr.	0 - 1 1/4 hr.	3/4 - 1 hr.
average	1/8 hr.	2/3 hr.	1 hr.
<u>Follow up</u>			
range	0 - 1 1/4 hrs.	0 - 3/4 hr.	1/2 hr.
average	1/8 hr.	1/4 hr.	1/2 hr.
<u>Total time</u>			
range	3/4-2 1/4 hrs.	1 1/2-5 1/4 hrs.	5 1/4-7 3/4 hrs.
average	1 1/3 hrs.	3 1/2 hrs.	7 hrs.

Abbott-Northwestern Hospital/ Sister Kenny Institute

800 East 28th Street
Minneapolis, MN 55407

Ellen Loux, OTR
Occupational Therapy Director
(612) 863-4447

Type of setting:
Rehabilitation (Inpatient and Outpatient)

Number of beds:
38

Total number of FTEs for this setting:
8.4

Productivity standard (in hours per day):
OTR Entry Level: 5.0 hrs.
OTR Inter. Level: 5.0-5.5 hrs.
OTR Adv. Level: N/A
COTA Entry Level: 5.0 hrs.
COTA Inter. Level: 5.0-5.6 hrs.
COTA Adv. Level: N/A
Manager/Director: 0 hrs.
Fieldwork Supervisor/Coordinator: 5.0 hrs.

Type of setting:
General Hospital

Number of beds:
720

Total number of FTEs for this setting:
2.7

Productivity standard (in hours per day):
OTR Entry Level: 4.5 hrs.
OTR Inter. Level: 4.5 hrs.
OTR Adv. Level: N/A
COTA Entry Level: N/A
COTA Inter. Level: 5.0 hrs.
COTA Adv. Level: N/A
Manager/Director: N/A

Continues on next page

This facility tracks productivity for the individual therapist and for the department as a whole, based on billable hours and required hours of work necessary to perform that amount of work. The generic standard is 5.0 hours per day, with specific standards set for different areas or programs as noted above. Each therapist is assigned to a specific team. However, everyone is cross-trained to work in multiple areas to accommodate census fluctuations.

To manage data appropriately, service codes are documented separately for inpatient/outpatient rehabilitation (SKI/OUTPT), brain injury clinic (BIC), acute care (ABBOTT-NORTHWESTERN), and cardiac rehabilitation (CORONARY REHAB) on **Form A**. The typical billable unit is 15 minutes, and the charge codes on this form are based on the CPT (Current Procedural Terminology), HCPCS (HCFA Common Procedural Coding System), and the Occupational Therapy Services table compiled by the Minnesota Occupational Therapy Association Reimbursement Committee.

Form B is a sample of an inpatient documentation record in which the therapist is to include length of treatment, reasons for cancellations, equipment issued, and any other pertinent information. Weekly notes are also done on this form, but the evaluation conference summary and progress and discharge notes are dictated separately. **Form C** is an outpatient documentation sheet that is completed for a month. Equipment issued is listed under each week for insurance purposes.

Form D is a Therapist TimeSheet that supplements the information generated on the Charge Ticket (**Form A**). **Attachment A** is a Monthly Productivity Summary that compares the department on a month-to-month basis.

All forms and attachments in this section are courtesy of Abbott-Northwestern Hospital/Sister Kenny Institute. Reprinted with permission.

Fieldwork Supervisor/Coordinator: N/A
Clinical Supervisor: 3.0 hrs.

Type of setting:
Cardiac Rehabilitation Unit

Number of beds:
137

Total number of FTEs for this setting:
7.8

Productivity standard (in hours per day):
OTR Entry Level: 4.2 hrs.
OTR Inter. Level: 4.2 hrs.
OTR Adv. Level: N/A
COTA Entry Level: 4.2 hrs.
COTA Inter. Level: 4.2 hrs.
COTA Adv. Level: N/A
Manager/Director: N/A
Fieldwork Supervisor/Coordinator: N/A
Clinical Supervisor: 3.0 hrs.

OCCUPATIONAL THERAPY

DATE ___ TIME ___ MODE ___ ORDER NO. ___

DIAGNOSIS/REASON ___

ORDER ___

EQUIPMENT ___

COST ___

REASON FOR CANCELLATION ___

Code	Description
0512	INITIAL VISIT
0514	SUBSEQUENT VISIT
0515	CANCELLATION
4166	INITIAL VISIT ORTHO
4340	SUBSEQUENT VISIT ORTHO
4345	INITIAL VISIT 25
4347	SUBSEQUENT VISIT 25
4396	INITIAL VISIT ONCOLOGY
4398	SUBSEQUENT VISIT ONCOLOGY
4401	INITIAL VISIT NEURO
4402	SUBSEQUENT VISIT NEURO
4540	INITIAL VISIT LOW BACK
4544	SUBSEQUENT VISIT LOW BACK
2221	EQUIPMENT
61136	NON-COVERED EQUIPMENT

CORONARY REHAB.

Code	Description
0530	COR. REHAB. EV. 15 MIN.
0527	COR. REHAB. EV. 30 MIN.
4843	COR. REHAB. I 15 MIN.
4068	COR. REHAB. I 30 MIN.
4840	COR. REHAB. II 15 MIN.
4841	COR. REHAB. II 30 MIN.
0548	COR. REHAB. III 15 MIN.
0549	COR. REHAB. III 30 MIN.
1906	COR. REHAB. ADL. EV. 15 MIN.
1907	COR. REHAB. ADL. EV. 30 MIN.
1909	COR. REHAB-ADL. TRNG 15
1910	COR. REHAB-ADL. TRNG 30
1918	COR. REHAB. HOME EVAL. 15
1920	COR. REHAB. HOME EVAL. 30
0553	COR. REHAB. INT. VISIT
0554	COR. REHAB. SUBVISIT

ABBOTT-NORTHWESTERN

Code	Description
0445	EVALUATION 15 MIN.
0447	EVALUATION 30 MIN.
63703	EVAL. ADD. 15 MIN.
0491	THERAPEUTIC EXERCISE 15 MIN.
0492	THERAPEUTIC EXERCISE 30 MIN.
63704	NEUROMUSCULAR RE-ED. 15 MIN.
63705	NEUROMUSCULAR RE-ED. 30 MIN.
63706	FUNCT. ACT. (GRP) 30 MIN.
63916	FUNCT. ACT. 1:1 15 MIN.
2795	FUNCT. ACT. 1:1 30 MIN.
63707	FA/NEURO/TE ADD. 15 MIN.
63708	KINETIC ACTIVITIES 15 MIN.
63709	KINETIC ACTIVITIES 30 MIN.
63710	KINETIC ACTIVITIES ADD. 15 MIN.
2790	ADL/HOMEMAKING 15 MIN.
2791	ADL/HOMEMAKING 30 MIN.
0486	THERA ORTHO. 15 MIN.
0487	THERA ORTHO. 30 MIN.
63711	ADL/THER. ADD. 15 MIN.
63712	TREATMENT 15 MIN. (B.I.)
0510	PT. CONF. 15 MIN.

BIC

Code	Description
61207	COMPENSATORY STRATEGY 15 MIN.
62518	BIC EVAL. 15 MIN.
63679	BIC PT. CONF. 15 MIN.
62521	BIC TX. (GRP) 15 MIN.
63682	BIC SUP. SKILL TRAINING 15 MIN.
63674	BIC INITIAL VISIT
63675	BIC SUBSEQUENT VISIT
63676	BIC CANCELLATION
63246	BIC EQUIPMENT
63247	BIC NON-COVERED EQUIP.

SKI/OUT PT.

Code	Description
1632	EVALUATION 15 MIN.
4838	EVALUATION 30 MIN.
63692	EVAL. ADD. 15 MIN.
4844	THERAPEUTIC EXERCISE 15 MIN.
5333	THERAPEUTIC EXERCISE 30 MIN.
63693	NEUROMUSCULAR RE-ED. 15 MIN.
63694	NEUROMUSCULAR RE-ED. 30 MIN.
0438	FUNCT. ACT. (GRP) 30 MIN.
63915	FUNCT. ACT. 1:1 15 MIN.
2783	FUNCT. ACT. 1:1 30 MIN.
63695	FA/NEURO/TE ADD. 15 MIN.
63696	KINETIC ACTIVITIES 15 MIN.
63697	KINETIC ACTIVITIES 30 MIN.
63698	KINETIC ACTIVITIES ADD. 15 MIN.
2781	ADL/HOMEMAKING EVAL. 15 MIN.
1850	ADL/HOMEMAKING EVAL. 30 MIN.
63699	ADL/HOMEMAKING EVAL. ADD. 15 MIN.
4839	ADL/HOMEMAKING TX. 15 MIN.
4871	ADL/HOMEMAKING TX. 30 MIN.
0192	THERA ORTHO. 15 MIN.
0196	THERA ORTHO. 30 MIN.

Code	Description
63700	ADL/THER. ADD. 15 MIN.
63701	TREATMENT 15 MIN. (B.I.)
4551	O.T. INDEP. LIVING SKILLS (GRP)
2788	SUP. SKILL TRAINING 15 MIN.
63319	EVAL./REEVAL LTC 15 MIN.
63320	SVCS-LTC 15 MIN. X 6005
7251	EVAL. CONF. 15 MIN.
7252	PROGRESS CONFERENCE 15 MIN.
0429	PT. CONF. 15 MIN.
5722	REHAB. ENG. 15 MIN.
63702	REHAB. ENG. ADD. TX. 15 MIN.
3855	INITIAL VISIT
3856	SUBSEQUENT VISIT
3857	CANCELLATION
2220	EQUIPMENT $
4230	NON-COVERED EQUIP.

DEFINITIONS FOR SERVICE CODES

THERAPEUTIC EXERCISE: Instructing a patient in exercises and directly supervising the exercises. Exercising done subsequently by the patient without a therapist present and supervising will not be covered by this code.

> **Treatment:** Instructing patients in self-ROM exercises, SROM, icing, home programs, home program preparation.

NEUROMUSCULAR RE-EDUCATION: Provision of direct services to a patient who has neuromuscular impairment and is undergoing recovery or regeneration. Examples would be surgery, trauma to neuromuscular system, cerebral vascular accident, and systemic neurological disease.

> **Treatment:** NDT, PNF, biofeedback, rhizotomies.

FUNCTIONAL ACTIVITIES: The development and instruction in specific activities for persons who are handicapped or debilitated by neuromusculoskeletal dysfunction. This applies to counseling and instructions in body mechanics and work-related activities.

> **Treatment:** All group charges, endurance group, functional group, technique group.

KINETIC ACTIVITIES: Services when there are neuromusculoskeletal dysfunction which limit the patient's performing the activities that are ordinarily prescribed under therapeutic exercise. To increase coordination, strength, and/or range of motion, one area (any two extremities or trunk).

> **Treatment:** PRE's, PROM, coordination, ergometer, cardiac calisthenics, strengthening activities, decongestive massage.

ACTIVITIES OF DAILY LIVING/ADL'S: Services provided to impaired individuals; for example, how to get in and out of a tub, how to make a bed, how to prepare a meal in a kitchen. Self-care skills and/or daily life management skills. Does not apply to instructions or counseling in body mechanics given to a patient.

> **Treatment:** Positioning, feeding group, kitchen, home program, energy conservation, joint protection, one-handed techniques, adapted equipment.

THERAPEUTIC ORTHOTICS: Orthotic training, mouthstick training, mobile arm support equipment, deltoid aide activities.

Not all brain injury treatment should go under BI 15 min. Look at other coding that may be appropriate; i.e., neuromuscular, ADLs.

Home visits are to be documented as EVALUATION.

BIC codes are specifically designed for the brain injury clinic and are all documented in 15-minute units.

CORONARY REHABILITATION:

1. Coronary Rehabilitation Evaluation: Includes chart review, contact with nursing, interview, and initial treatment to determine baseline data.

2. Coronary Rehabilitation I: One-on-one with patient in room, including treatment and home program.

3. Coronary Rehabilitation II: Two or more patients treated in the clinic.

4. Coronary Rehabilitation III: Group setting for work equivalent activity, work simplification, education, and supportive treatment.

5. ADL Evaluation: Activities of daily living evaluation performed in patient's room. This usually includes light hygiene, bathing, grooming, feeding, and dressing, as appropriate.

6. ADL Training: Training in any of the areas listed above.

7. Homemaking Evaluation: Evaluation of homemaking skills, such as light meal preparation and light cleaning.

**ABBOTT-NORTHWESTERN HOSPITAL CORPORATION
SISTER KENNY INSTITUTE**
800 E. 28th St. at Chicago Ave.
Minneapolis, MN 55407

SKI—INPATIENT RECORD TREATMENT & TIME

Patient Name _____ Date _____

DAY	MONDAY				TUESDAY				WEDNESDAY				THURSDAY				FRIDAY				SAT.		SUN.
DATE																							
STUDENT SUPERVISOR																							
THERAPIST																							
EVALUATION																							
THERAPEUTIC EXERCISE																							
NEUROMUSC. RE-ED.																							
FUNCT. ACT (GROUP)																							
FUNCT. ACT 1:1																							
KINETIC ACTIVITIES																							
A.D.L.'S																							
HOMEMAKING																							
THERAPEUTIC ORTHOTICS																							
TREATMENT (B.I.)																							
INDEP. LIVING SKILLS																							
SUPERVISED SKILL TRG.																							
TEAM CONFERENCE																							
PATIENT CONFERENCE																							
REASON FOR CANCELLATION																							

EQUIPMENT: _____

COMMENTS: _____
_____
_____
_____
_____
_____
_____

OCCUPATIONAL THERAPY

MMC 353C
65-17670

OCCUPATIONAL THERAPY

Out Patient
ABBOTT-NORTHWESTERN HOSPITAL CORPORATION
SISTER KENNY INSTITUTE
800 E. 28th St. at Chicago Ave.
Minneapolis, MN 55407

PROGRESS NOTE: Daily Attendance
and Weekly Summaries

NAME: _____

SOCIAL SECURITY #: _____

PHYSICIAN: _____

INSURANCE: _____

Monthly Short Term Goals: _____

Attendance:

Date:

Time Seen:

M T W TH F | M T W TH F | M T W TH F | M T W TH F

Equipment issued:
_____ Patient was informed
that insurance company may
not cover equipent
and agreed to pay.

Monthly Note and
plan dictated
Date _____

_____ Continue. Please refer to monthly summary for
revised goals and time frame.
_____ Discontinue. Please refer to dischnrge summary

_____, OTR

_____, OTR

OCCUPATIONAL THERAPY

Key: L=Late NS=No Show C=Cancelled

O-1

65-71536

OCCUPATIONAL THERAPY

Form D

ABBOTT NORTHWESTERN HOSPITAL

a LifeSpan® member

800 E. 28TH ST AT CHICAGO AVE.
MINNEAPOLIS MINNESOTA 55407
PHONE 612/863-4000

MONTH

NAME

	REGULAR HOURS	COVERAGE	EXTRA COVERAGE	PTO	ADMIN	EDUCATION	ORIENTATION	COMP EARNED	COMP USED	*STUDENT HOURS	BILLED SKI	BILLED ACUTE	BILLED O.P.	BILLED BIC	GROUP HOURS	HRS. CANC. SKI	HRS. CANC. ACUTE	HRS. CANC. O.P.	HRS CANC. BIC	*NO TIMES	PT. DELAY <15'	*RDS/MTGS	Q.A.	PROGRAM DEVEL.	*OTS
1																									
2																									
3																									
4																									
5																									
6																									
7																									
8																									
9																									
10																									
11																									
12																									
13																									
14																									
15																									
16																									
17																									
18																									
19																									
20																									
21																									
22																									
23																									
24																									
25																									
26																									
27																									
28																									
29																									
30																									
31																									

* STUDENT HOURS = Direct Hours of student treatment

NO TIMES = Number of treatments unable to schedule due to time constraints

RDS/MTG = Time spent on rounds and SCI, CVA, BI, BIC meetings, including orientation of staff

OTS = Time spent managing students

TIME SHEETS

Regular Hours: permanent staff either full or part time
                  hours or staff replacing floated to position
                  i.e. cardiac, work injury

Coverage Hours: filling in for a specific person

Extra Coverage: additional staff because of increased
                  caseload, not replacing anyone

PTO: Vacation or Sick (ill) time designated by hours and
                  letter i.e. 8I, 8V

Education: time spent in workshops or inservice time
                  for coverage therapist.

Orientation: time spent in orientation to department

Administration: supervisor's non-patient treatment time,
                  OTR's performing supervisory duties.

Comp earned/used: 30 min. increments

Student Hours: direct hours of students treatment

Billed SKI/O.P./ACUTE/BIC: 1:1 treatment charges. Day
                  Hospital hours are O.P.

Group Hours: therapist's time in group treatment/ 3 patients
                  or more

HRS SKI, acute, OP, BIC: hours of cancellations, include also
                  15 min. delays

No Time: number of treatments unable to schedule because of
                  time constraints

Patient Delays: anything under 15 min. of waiting;
                  time vs. #'s

Rds.\mtgs: attendance at stations rounds, SCI, CVA, BI, BIC
                  meetings. Do NOT include departmental staff or
                  team meetings. Include orientation time of staff.

Q.A.:

Program Development

OTS: time spent managing students including orientation,
consultation, patient observation, student preparation,
review of documentation etc.

ABBOTT NORTHWESTERN HOSPITAL
PRODUCTIVITY ENHANCEMENT PROGRAM

Page:

COST CENTER PRODUCTIVITY SUMMARY REPORT
PERIOD: 2 -

ORGANIZATION: ABBOTT - NORTHWESTERN   HOSPITAL: 1-ABBOTT - NORTHWESTERN
DIVISION:
DEPARTMENT: COST CENTER: 7530-Occupational Therapy

		ACTUAL					FTE'S				FTE VARIANCE	
PERIOD	TOTAL REQ HOURS	TOTAL WORKED HOURS*	OVER- TIME HOURS	PAID NON-WRKD SVH	TOTAL PAID HOURS	PROD INDEX	REQ WORKED#	REQ PAID#	ACTUAL PAID	BUDGET FTE'S	REQ-PD TO ACT-PD#	BUDGET TO ACT-PD

COST CENTER - HISTORICAL
        YEAR 1
        YEAR 2
        YEAR 3

COST CENTER - CURRENT YEAR

 1 - 01/01/90 TO 01/31/90
 2 - 02/01/90 TO 02/28/90

        Y-T-D
        AVERAGE

COST CENTER - LABOR COST

 CURRENT PERIOD COST ($)
 Y-T-D AVERAGE COST ($)
 Y-T-D TOTAL COST   ($)

   * INCLUDES OVERTIME HOURS
   # FTE'S CALCULATED AT 100% PRODUCTIVITY

CURRENT PERIOD PRODUCTIVITY INDEX*

                                          ****
CUMULATIVE PRODUCTIVITY INDEX   *   *
                                          ****

PRODUCTIVITY GOAL   0.0 TO   0.0

                    TOTAL REQUIRED HOURS
 * PRODUCTIVITY INDEX = ------------------------------------- X 100
                    ACTUAL HOURS (INCLUDING OVERTIME)

Managing Productivity in Occupational Therapy

```
DATE                              ABBOTT NORTHWESTERN HOSPITAL                    Page:
TIME                              PRODUCTIVITY ENHANCEMENT PROGRAM


                                  COST CENTER PRODUCTIVITY DETAIL REPORT
                                      PERIOD: 2 -


ORGANIZATION:  ABBOTT - NORTHWESTERN           HOSPITAL:      1-ABBOTT - NORTHWESTERN
DIVISION:
DEPARTMENT:                                    COST CENTER:   7530-Occupational Therapy


                        PERSON                                                    CURRENT     YTD
                         HOUR  |_____WORKLOAD UNIT VOLUME_____|          PRD REQ   AVERAGE
WORKLOAD UNIT          STANDARD    PERIOD: 1      2                               PERSON HRS  VOLUME
==========================================================================================================
 BILLABLE HOURS
--------------------------------------------------------------------------------------------------------
RATIOS:

 WORKED HOURS/ADJUSTED PT. DAYS
 WORKED DOLLARS/BILLABLE HOURS
 WORKED HOUR/BILLABLE HOUR
 WRKD HRS/ADJ DISC


==========================================================================================================
==========================================================================================================
```

```
                                       TOTAL REQUIRED HOURS
                                       ACTUAL WKD PERSON HOURS

                                                                    ********
                                       CURRENT PERIOD PRODUCTIVITY INDEX*   *        *
                                                                    ********

                                       CUMULATIVE PRODUCTIVITY INDEX

                                       PRODUCTIVITY GOAL               TO

                                       REQUIRED FTE'S
                                       ACTUAL WKD FTE'S


                             TOTAL REQUIRED HOURS
        * PRODUCTIVITY INDEX = ------------------------------------ X 100
                             ACTUAL HOURS (INCLUDING OVERTIME)
```

Abbott-Northwestern Hospital/Sister Kenny Institute

Henry Ford Hospital

2799 West Grand Boulevard
Detroit, MI 48202-2689

Sheila Mack, MS, OTR
Director of Occupational Therapy
(313) 876-1127

Type of setting:
General Hospital/Teaching Facility

Number of beds:
900

Total number of FTEs for this setting:
16
1 Director
12 OTRs
2 COTAs
1 Secretary

Productivity standard (in hours per day):
OTR Entry Level: 5.0-6.0 hrs.
OTR Inter. Level: 5.0-6.0 hrs.
OTR Adv. Level: 4.0-5.0 hrs.
COTA Entry Level: 5.0-6.0 hrs.
COTA Inter. Level: 5.0-6.0 hrs.
COTA Adv. Level: N/A
Manager/Director: 0 hrs.
Fieldwork Supervisor/Coordinator:1.5-2.0 hrs.

Type of setting:
Work Hardening Program (off site)

Number of beds:
N/A

Total number of FTEs for this setting:
4
2 OTRs
1 COTA
1 Secretary

T his facility uses 15-minute intervals as its billable units of time (BUT). They also track nonbillable units of time (NBUT) and include that in their productivity standard. Examples of NBUT are: team or vendor meetings; time spent with school therapists to discuss a patient referral; or when two OTs see one patient at the same time (e.g., to make a complicated splint).

In addition to the productivity standard by hours and units of time noted above, they also have established staff-patient ratios as follows:

- Physical Dysfunction:
  1 to 5 patients = .5 OTR
  6 to 10 patients = 1.0 OTR

- Return to Work:
  0 to 5 clients = 1.0 OTR
  6 to 10 clients = 2.0 OTR
  10 to 13 clients = 2.5 OTR & COTA
  13 to 15 clients = 3.0 OTR & COTA
  15 to 20 clients = 4.0 OTR & COTA

- Psychiatry
  1 to 10 patients = 1.0 OTR
  11 to 15 patients = 1.5 OTR
  16 to 20 patients = 2.0 OTR
  21 to 25 patients = 2.5 OTR
  26 to 30 patients = 3.0 OTR
  31 to 35 patients = 3.5 OTR

Forms A, B, and C are the weekly, monthly, and yearly reporting sheets/reports. **Form D** is the Occupational Therapy Billing Sheet. (Note that RTWC is the Return to Work Center.)

All forms in this section are courtesy of Henry Ford Hospital, Occupational Therapy Department, Detroit, MI. Reprinted with permission.

Continues on next page

Productivity standard (in hours per day):
OTR Entry Level: 6.0 hrs.
OTR Inter. Level: 6.0 hrs.
OTR Adv. Level: 4.5 hrs.
COTA Entry Level: 6.0 hrs.
COTA Inter. Level: 6.0 hrs..
COTA Adv. Level: N/A
Manager/Director: N/A
Fieldwork Supervisor/Coordinator: N/A
Supervisor: 4.5 hrs.

Type of setting:
Mental Health Unit in General Hospital/Teaching Facility

Number of beds:
16

Total number of FTEs for this setting:
1.5

Productivity standard (in hours per day):
OTR Entry Level: 6.0 hrs.
OTR Inter. Level: 6.0 hrs.
OTR Adv. Level (Senior OTR position): 5.0 hrs.
COTA Entry Level: N/A
COTA Inter. Level: N/A
COTA Adv. Level: N/A
Manager/Director: N/A
Fieldwork Supervisor/Coordinator: N/A

NAME: _____

WEEK OF: _____

HENRY FORD HOSPITAL
OT DEPT – PHYS. DYS.
WEEKLY STAT SHEETS

DIRECT BILL. PATIENT CARE	MONDAY			TUESDAY			WEDNESDAY			THURSDAY			FRIDAY			SATURDAY			TOTALS		
	#OF Pts	DPC	BUT	#OF Pts	DPC	BUT	#OF Pts	DPC	BUT	#OF Pts	DPC	BUT	#OF Pts	DPC	BUT	#OF Pts	DPC	BUT	#OF Pts	DPC	BUT
IN-PATIENT ORTHO																					
OUT-Pt. ORTHO PLASTIC CLINIC																					
NONBILL. ORTHO IN-PATIENT																					
NONBILL. ORTHO OUT-PATIENT																					
IN-PATIENT NEURO																					
OUT-PATIENT NEURO																					
NONBILL. NEURO IN-PATIENT																					
NONBILL. NEURO OUT-PATIENT																					
IN-PATIENT PEDS																					
OUT-PATIENT PEDS																					
NONBILL. PEDS IN-PATIENT																					
NONBILL. PEDS OUT-PATIENT																					
IN-PATIENT NEPHRO																					
NONBILL. NEPH. IN-PATIENT																					
NONBILL. NEPH OUT_PATIENT																					
ALS CLINIC																					
CARDI CLASS																					

	MONDAY	TUESDAY	WEDNESDAY	THURSDAY	FRIDAY	SATURDAY	TOTALS
IN-DIRECT PATIENT CARE	IPC	IPC	IPC	IPC	IPC	IPC	IPC
MDC/PLASTICS DOWN TIME							
ROUNDS TEAM CONFERENCE							
SENIOR STAFF							
STAFF MEETINGS							
INSERVICES							
STUDENT SUPERVISION							
ADMINISTRATION MISC.							
TOTALS							

HENRY FORD HOSPITAL

OT PSYCH_____

OCCUPATIONAL THERAPY DEPARTMENT   Month_____ Year_____

OT RTWC_____

MONTHLY STATISTICAL REPORT

OT PHYS DYS_____

DATE (WEEKS)

EMPLOYEE	DATA							TOTAL	% OF PROD.
1.	# Pt. DPC								
	BUT								
	Hr. Wk								
	# Pt. NBUT DPC								
	Dr. Rounds Dr. ↓								
2.	# Pt DPC								
	BUT								
	Hr. Wk								
	# Pt. NBUT DPC								
	Dr. Rounds Dr. ↓								
3.	# Pt. DPC								
	BUT								
	Hr. Wk								
	# Pt. NBUT DPC								
	Dr. Rounds Dr ↓								

END OF MONTH STATS:

TOTALS:

        # Pts Tx_____

        # DPC Time_____

        # BUT_____

        # NBUT_____

        # NB DPC_____

        # Dr Rounds_____

        # Dr ↓ _____

        # Emp Hrs Wk_____

HENRY FORD HOSPITAL
OCCUPATIONAL THERAPY DEPARTMENT
STATISTICAL REPORT

YEAR: _____

VOLUME STATISTICS - PHYSICAL DYSFUNCTION #204570	JAN	FEB	MAR	APR	MAY	JUNE	JULY	AUG	SEPT	OCT	NOV	DEC	TOTAL
NEURO: # of IP													
# of IP Contacts													
# of IP BUT													
# of OP													
# of OP Contacts													
# of OP BUT													
ORTHO: # of IP													
# of IP Contacts													
# of IP BUT													
# of OP													
# of OP Contacts													
# of OP BUT													
PEDS: # of IP													
# of IP Contacts													
# of IP BUT													
# of OP													
# of OP Contacts													
# of OP BUT													
NEPHRO: # of IP													
# of IP Contacts													
# of IP BUT													
CARDI CLASS (IP) # of IP Contacts													
# of BUT													
TOTALS: IP CONTACTS													
OP CONTACTS													
IP BUT													
OP BUT													

HENRY FORD HOSPITAL
OCCUPATIONAL THERAPY DEPARTMENT
STATISTICAL REPORT

VOLUME STATISTICS – PHYSICAL DYSFUNCTION #204570	JAN	FEB	MAR	APR	MAY	JUNE	JULY	AUG	SEPT	OCT	NOV	DEC	TOTAL
# of New Referrals to the Dept.													
# of Discont./discharges from the Dept.													
# of Cancellations/No Shows (Dept/Pt)													
# of Days of Treatment													
# of FTE's (Support/patient treatment)													
DRS MTGS/ROUNDS #/UT													
BILLED REVENUE													

VOLUME STATISTICS – RTWC #204566	JAN	FEB	MAR	APR	MAY	JUNE	JULY	AUG	SEPT	OCT	NOV	DEC	TOTAL
# of New Referrals Open/pending													
# of Discharges (Closed Cases) WH/other													
# of Evaluations Total/eval only													
# of Eval. BUT Total/eval only													
# of Screenings Re-eval/screen only													
# of Screening BUT Total/screen only													
# of Work Hardening Clients													
# of Work Hardening Contacts													
# of Work Hardening BUT's													
# of On Job Site Contacts													
# of On Job Site BUT's													
Total # of Clients (W.H., Eval, Screening)													
Total # of BUT (W.H., Eval, Screening)													
# of Cancellations Pt/Dept.													
# of Days of Treatment													
# of FTE's													
BILLED REVENUE													

OCCUPATIONAL THERAPY DEPARTMENT
STATISTICAL REPORT

PHYSICAL DYSFUNCTION
PERSONNEL PRODUCTIVITY STATISTICS:

	JAN	FEB	MAR	APR	MAY	JUNE	JULY	AUG	SEPT	OCT	NOV	DEC	AVG. TOTALS
SUPERVISING OTR													
OTR													
OTR													
OTR													
OTR													
OTR													
OTR													
OTR													
OTR													
OTR													
OTR													
OTR													
OTR													
STUDENT													
STUDENT													
STUDENT													
STUDENT													
STUDENT													
STUDENT													
STUDENT													
STUDENT													
COTA													
COTA													
COTA													
RELIEF/CONTINGENT													
RELIEF/CONTINGENT													

FTE =

HENRY FORD HOSPITAL
OCCUPATIONAL THERAPY DEPARTMENT
STATISTICAL REPORT

RETURN TO WORK CENTER PERSONNEL PRODUCTIVITY STATISTICS:	JAN	FEB	MAR	APR	MAY	JUNE	JULY	AUG	SEPT	OCT	NOV	DEC	AVG. TOTAL
SUPERVISING OTR													
OTR													
OTR													
OTR													
OTR													
OTR													
STUDENT													
STUDENT													
STUDENT													
COTA													
COTA													
RELIEF/CONTINGENT													

DEPARTMENT TOTAL PII

Average Units Per Day Per Services

Phys. Dys.   =   (17)

RTWC   =   (28)

Dept. Total   =   (22.5)

DEPT. FTE: OT PAYS #

OTHER PAYS #

BUDGETED #

DEPT. TOTAL REVENUE:

ℋℯ𝓃𝓇𝓎 ℱℴ𝓇𝒹 ℋℴ𝓈𝓅𝒾𝓉𝒶𝓁

OCCUPATIONAL THERAPY BILLING SHEET

Form 97-3 Rev 6/91

DAILY STATISTICAL INFORMATION

Ortho/Plast_____ Peds_____ Neuro_____ Nephro_____ Cardi_____ RTWC_____

Date/Day:_____

Name:_____

Hrs. Worked:_____ x 4UT = _____

New
Ref #_____

Pt.
Cancel #_____

IPD: BUT:_____ Contacts_____ DPC_____

         NBUT:_____ Contacts_____ DPC_____

OPD: BUT:_____ Contacts_____ DPC_____

         NBUT:_____ Contacts_____ DPC_____

Dept.
Cancel #_____

Discharge #_____

DR. Rounds: #_____ UT_____

DR. Down UT:_____ Misc/Mtg. UT_____

COST CENTERS
(circle one)

204566	314570
204570	304570
204571	

TIME	MRN	SUFFIX	ADM. DATE	PT. NAME	INSUR	DX CODE OR RM #

Managing Productivity in Occupational Therapy

PT. STAT. INFO.						PHYSICAL DYSFUNCTION																							RTWC				CLINICS				Functional Training Classes		
ONGOING PATIENT	NEW PATIENT	SAME DAY WALK IN	D/C	PT. UNAV/NO SHOW/CANCEL	DEPT. CANCEL	439012 F.O.P.D. CAID EVAL 0/30	439014 F.O.P.D. CAID EVAL 31/60	439204 F.O.P.D. CAID PROC M&C	43902(4) Evaluation	43923(4) Graded ROM Act	43924(4) PRE/ISOM Act	43926(4) NEURO PHIS	43931(4) Motor Coor Act	43930(4) Developmental Act	43927(4) Transfer Act	43940(4) Cog/Percep Act	43936(4) ADL Training	43937(4) EngCon/WkSim	43932(4) Home Program	43939(4) Sensory Act	43925(4) Stretching Act	43946(1) Edema Control	43941(4) Scar Massage	43944(4) Thermo Treatment Act	43906(4) Splint Fabrication	909007 Splint Fab 1X BC	77951 Equipment	77961 Equipment PtPay	43905 Evaluation	43910 Work Hardening	43908 Dis Sum	43909 Home Program	43906 Job Site	43907 Screening	43970(4) MDC Clinic	43971(4) DAC Clinic	43972(4) ALS Clinic	43973(4) MYELO Clinic	43980(4) Cardiac Class	43982(4) Stress Mgt	43983(4) Undefined

National Rehabilitation Hospital

102 Irving Street, N.W.
Washington, DC 20010

Dianne McCarthy, MS, OTR/L
Director of Occupational Therapy
Deborah Lieberman, MHSA, OTR/L
Consultant
(202) 877-1531

Type of setting:
Rehabilitation Hospital

Number of beds:
160

Total number of FTEs for this setting:
66.5 (inpatient and outpatient)
Management: 9 (OTRs)
Senior OTRs: 14.5 (OTRs)
Staff: 28 (OTRs)
Assistants: 3 (COTAs)
Aides: 8
Office Staff: 4

Productivity standard (in hours per day):
OTR Entry Level: 6.5 hrs. (inpatient)
OTR Inter. Level: 6.5 hrs. (inpatient)
OTR Adv. Level: 6.0 hrs. (inpatient)
COTA Entry Level: 6.5 hrs. (inpatient)
COTA Inter. Level: 6.5 hrs. (inpatient)
COTA Adv. Level: 6.5 hrs. (inpatient)
Manager/Director: 0 hrs.
Fieldwork Supervisor/Coordinator: 0 hrs.
OT Aides: None established

In February 1991, this 160-bed rehabilitation hospital underwent a conversion to a computerized charge capture system through the use of bar-code charge codes. This is part of a hospitalwide implementation of a Management Information System.

Productivity can be evaluated on an individual, program, team, and servicewide basis, with the capability to differentiate between inpatient and outpatient programs. The overall charging and documentation system is based on AOTA's *Product Output Reporting System and Uniform Terminology for Reporting Occupational Therapy Services (first edition)*. Productivity is currently evaluated in terms of billable units and intensity of treatment (RVUs). As the system develops, productivity will also include daily contact hours. One unit of service equals 15 minutes. The budgeted productivity standard is 6.5 contact hours per therapist per 8.5-hour day.

The system incorporates use of the following attached forms:

Attachment A—Patient Schedule

This form shows the patient's activities for the day. It includes the time, the therapist, the service (discipline), and the location of the treatment. The schedule reflects individual, group, and cotreatments. It also includes some demographic information, hospital number, diagnosis, and physician.

The patient schedule serves as the basis for generating computerized bar-coded charge tickets. An individual charge ticket (Attachment B) is generated for each scheduled treatment.

Attachment B—Charge Ticket

Bar-coded charge tickets are generated for each scheduled treatment and distributed to the assigned therapist. The therapist manually fills in the quantity or number of units provided upon completion of the therapy session. The bar-coded information is then entered into the computer system by support staff using a bar-code wand.

The bar codes for each service category contain the unit value and the associated rate. This figure multiplied by the quantity equals the charge and RVU. Side 2 of Attachment B contains additional charges

Continues on next page

as well as codes to record lost time. Therapists document the number of time units (quantity) scheduled but not provided. This information is then generated into a separate lost time report (Attachment E).

Attachment C—Weekly Productivity Report by Therapist

This report reflects the number of time units and associated revenue generated on a daily basis per therapist. Comparison with productivity requirements varies, depending on the therapist's employment status, schedule, number of work hours, etc.

Attachment D—Weekly Productivity Report by Team

Information from individual therapists assigned to specific teams/programs is grouped together in this report. These team reports are distributed and reviewed by the team supervisor for comments and follow-up.

Attachment E—Weekly Lost Time Report

As noted under the explanation for Attachment B, the therapist documents reasons why scheduled therapy was not provided. This report summarizes these data by nursing unit. This report can then be used to identify specific unit problems and plans for correction.

Attachment F—Monthly Summary by Team

This report summarizes information from the Weekly Productivity Report (Attachment D) on a monthly basis.

Attachment G—Exception Report (Reconciliation Report)

This report itemizes those computer generated tickets that could not be accounted for at the end of business. It is generated on a daily basis. Support staff follow up with the respective therapist to ensure that all charges were submitted and all scheduled treatment can be accounted for within the system.

Attachment H—Documentation Record

This is an example of a proposed weekly documentation record that would correspond directly with the daily charge ticket. The record is generated by the patient and includes information regarding the type of service provided, the therapist (by code), and the number of time units (quantity). It is being proposed that some type of report similar to this format will become part of the medical record.

All attachments in this section are courtesy of National Rehabilitation Hospital, Washington, DC. Reprinted with permission.

MONDAY, JUNE 10, 1991   2 EAST

3:22 PM   ROOMS 214-1 — 217-1

Patient Name Room # Patient No. Diagnosis Physician	Patient Name Room # Patient No. Diagnosis Physician	Patient Name Room # Patient No. Diagnosis Physician	Patient Name Room # Patient No. Diagnosis Physician	
2 FLOOR MEAL TIMES	**2 FLOOR MEAL TIMES**	**2 FLOOR MEAL TIMES**	**2 FLOOR MEAL TIMES**	
7:00 BREAKFST	BREAKFST	BREAKFST	BREAKFST	7:00
7:15 BREAKFST	BREAKFST	BREAKFST	BREAKFST	7:15
7:30 BREAKFST	BREAKFST	BREAKFST	BREAKFST	7:30
7:45 BREAKFST	BREAKFST	BREAKFST	BREAKFST	7:45
8:00			OTMAGUIR BS/DLS	8:00
8:15			OTMAGUIR BS/DLS	8:15
8:30				8:30
8:45				8:45
9:00	OTVERONI OT			9:00
9:15	OTVERONI OT			9:15
9:30 PTMEEHAN PT TF	OTVERONI OT	*FAS/GRP2 OT		9:30
9:45 PTMEEHAN PT TF	OTVERONI OT	FAS/GRP2 OT		9:45
10:00 PSY/CVA CHAPEL	PYCVACHE 2W CONF R	SPHALPER SP	AMPOOL1 PT	10:00
10:15 PSY/CVA CHAPEL	PYCVACHE 2W CONF R	SPHALPER SP	AMPOOL1 PT	10:15
10:30 PSY/CVA CHAPEL	PYCVACHE 2W CONF R		AMPOOL1 PT	10:30
10:45 PSY/CVA CHAPEL	PYCVACHE 2W CONF R		AMPOOL1 PT	10:45
11:00 PTWARD PT	FAM CONF FAM CONF	PY/CVA2 CHAPEL		11:00
11:15 PTWARD PT	FAM CONF FAM CONF	PY/CVA2 CHAPEL		11:15
11:30	FAM CONF FAM CONF	PY/CVA2 CHAPEL	OTMAGUIR OT	11:30
11:45	FAM CONF FAM CONF	PY/CVA2 CHAPEL	OTMAGUIR OT	11:45
12:00 LUNCH	LUNCH	LUNCH	LUNCH	12:00
12:15 LUNCH	LUNCH	LUNCH	LUNCH	12:15
12:30 LUNCH	LUNCH	LUNCH	LUNCH	12:30
12:45 LUNCH	LUNCH	LUNCH	LUNCH	12:45
1:00 OTKALTER OT		OTHUDSON OT	PTMEEHAN PT	1:00
1:15 OTKALTER OT		OTHUDSON OT	PTMEEHAN PT	1:15
1:30 OTKALTER OT	MCGROUPA 2E TREATM	AMBULATE 2EA	AMBULATE 2EA	1:30
1:45 OTKALTER OT	MCGROUPA 2E TREATM	AMBULATE 2EA	AMBULATE 2EA	1:45
2:00	MCGROUPA 2E TREATM	AMBULATE 2EA	AMBULATE 2EA	2:00
2:15	MCGROUPA 2E TREATM	AMBULATE 2EA	AMBULATE 2EA	2:15
2:30			SPHALPER SP	2:30
2:45			SPHALPER SP	2:45
3:00 *OTPSYGRO 3 WEST AT *		PYKORYTN RM 252	OTMAGUIR OT	3:00
3:15 OTPSYGRO 3 WEST AT		PYKORYTN RM 252	OTMAGUIR OT	3:15
3:30 OTPSYGRO 3 WEST AT	OTVERONI OT	PYKORYTN RM 252	PTMEEHAN PT	3:30
3:45 OTPSYGRO 3 WEST AT	OTVERONI OT	PYKORYTN RM 252	PTMEEHAN PT	3:45
4:00 PTMEEHAN PT TF	VRWILEY VR			4:00
4:15 PTMEEHAN PT TF	VRWILEY VR			4:15
4:30	VRWILEY VR	PTGALLEL PT		4:30
4:45	VRWILEY VR	PTGALLEL PT		4:45
5:00 DINNER	DINNER	DINNER	DINNER	5:00
5:15 DINNER	DINNER	DINNER	DINNER	5:15
5:30 DINNER	DINNER	DINNER	DINNER	5:30
5:45 DINNER	DINNER	DINNER	DINNER	5:45
6:00				6:00
6:15	* = OT Group			6:15
6:30				6:30
6:45				6:45

DEPT 210 OCCUPATIONAL THERAPY SERVICE DELIVERY FORM

PATIENT NUMBER	THERAPIST CODE	SERVICE DATE	CONTROL	THERAPIST INITIALS	GROUP NUMBER
9105016	Therapist A	060791	112	TIME OF SERVICE	

ASSESSMENTS	QTY	TREATMENT	QTY	SENS. MOTOR	QTY	COGNITIVE	QTY	PSYCHOSOC.	QTY
SCREEN 21001		PHYS 1 21134		NEURO REFL–INTG 21282		ORIENT 1 21415		SELF MGMT 21506	
CONSUL 21019		PHYS 21142		NEURO ROM 1 21290		ORIENT 21423		DYADIC INT 21530	
EVAL IL/DLS 21027		FUNC MOB 1 22090		NEURO ROM 21308		CONCEPT/COMP 1 21449		GROUP INT 21563	
EVAL SEN/MOT 21043		FUNC MOB 22108		NEURO COORD 1 21324		CONCEPT/COMP 21456		THER AD	QTY
EVAL COG 21068		COMM SK GP 1–3 22074		NEURO COORD 21332		INTEG 1 21472		ORTHO 21597	
EVAL THER AD 21084		COMM SK GP 4–6 22082		NEURO STR/END 1 21357		INTEG 21480		PROS 21621	
EVAL SPEC 21100		HOME MGT. 1 22116		NEURO STR/END 21365				ASSIST/ADAPT 21654	
EVAL DRIV 22066		HOME MGT. 22124		SENS INTEG 1 21381					
REASS 21118		WK/EMP 1 21225		SENS INTEG 21399					
		WK/EMP 21233							
		DRIV TRAIN 22173							

NRH
NATIONAL
REHABILITATION
HOSPITAL

Patient Number
Patient Name
Date of Birth
Admission Date
Physician

DEPT 210 OCCUPATIONAL THERAPY SERVICE DELIVERY FORM

PREVENTION	QTY	SPLINTING	QTY	ASSIST/ADAPT	QTY	OTHER CODES	QTY	LOST TIME	QTY
ENERGY CONS 1 ‖‖‖ 22132		UNIT 1 ‖‖‖ 21738		UNIT 1 ‖‖‖ 21779		CONFERENCE ‖‖‖ 21712		NO-SHOW ‖‖‖ 90014	
ENERGY CONS ‖‖‖ 22140		UNIT 2 ‖‖‖ 21746		UNIT 2 ‖‖‖ 21787		F.E.S. ‖‖‖ 20185		LATE ‖‖‖ 90022	
JT PROT/BD MECH ‖‖‖ 22157		UNIT 3 ‖‖‖ 21753		UNIT 3 ‖‖‖ 21795		F.E.S. RNT ‖‖‖ 20375		REFUSE ‖‖‖ 90030	
		UNIT 4 ‖‖‖ 21761		UNIT 4 ‖‖‖ 21803		TNS ‖‖‖ 20193		SICK ‖‖‖ 90048	
						TNS RNT ‖‖‖ 20367		SCH. CONFLICT ‖‖‖ 90055	
						EXT PUMP ‖‖‖ 22165		TESTING ‖‖‖ 90063	
						CO-TREAT(1) ‖‖‖ 99916		TREAT INTERRUPT ‖‖‖ 90071	
						CO-TREAT(GRP) ‖‖‖ 99924		SELF TRANSPORT ‖‖‖ 90089	
						HOME ‖‖‖ 99932		CANCEL THERAPY ‖‖‖ 90097	
						COMMUNITY ‖‖‖ 99940		CANCEL TRANS ‖‖‖ 90105	
								CANCEL PATIENT ‖‖‖ 90113	

5/29/'91

NATIONAL REHABILITATION HOSPITAL

OCCUPATION THERAPY PRODUCTIVITY REPORT

FOR PERIOD ENDING   05/26/91
SORTED BY THERAPIST NAME

TEST DATA

THERAPIST NAME	MON TOTAL UNITS / REVENUE	TUE	WED	THR	FRI	SAT	TOTALS
A	$1,211.04	$358.30	$934.37	$605.50	$830.04	$0.00	$3,939.25
B	22 / $762.00	38 / $1,081.77	18 / $580.55	22 / $671.24	35 / $970.67	$0.00	135 / $4,066.23
C	30 / $802.80	33 / $1,027.36	40 / $1,065.88	49 / $1,288.14	33 / $836.84	$0.00	185 / $5,021.02
D	14 / $412.72	31 / $900.36	17 / $569.20	28 / $709.84	14 / $412.72	$0.00	104 / $3,004.84
E	36 / $884.50	33 / $1,004.68	39 / $1,124.92	$0.00	36 / $1,045.48	$0.00	144 / $4,059.58
F	30 / $775.60	12 / $353.76	12 / $353.76	19 / $560.12	12 / $353.76	$0.00	85 / $2,397.00
G	32 / $576.88	$0.00	$0.00	$0.00	16 / $532.94	$0.00	48 / $1,109.82
H	28 / $1,095.42	18 / $610.05	33 / $1,113.51	44 / $1,233.72	62 / $1,710.00	$0.00	185 / $5,762.70
I	8 / $367.42	14 / $508.00	6 / $176.88	14 / $548.84	8 / $263.06	$0.00	50 / $1,864.20
J	48 / $1,301.80	34 / $1,052.34	17 / $507.99	36 / $918.48	48 / $1,360.74	$0.00	183 / $5,141.35
K	29 / $841.38	15 / $485.31	30 / $909.42	16 / $510.25	28 / $1,047.76	$0.00	118 / $3,794.12
L	$0.00	$0.00	16 / $501.18	16 / $562.40	20 / $707.54	$0.00	52 / $1,771.12
M	21 / $721.18	26 / $911.64	18 / $598.68	24 / $861.76	30 / $1,025.06	$0.00	119 / $4,118.32
	18 / $603.24	36 / $918.92	22 / $501.62	13 / $374.18	$0.00	$0.00	89 / $2,397.96

Managing Productivity in Occupational Therapy

5/29/91

NATIONAL REHABILITATION HOSPITAL
OCCUPATION THERAPY PRODUCTIVITY REPORT
FOR PERIOD ENDING 05/26/91
SUMMARY REPORT

WEEKLY SUMMARY

TEST DATA

TEAM	TOTAL UNITS / REVENUE	MON	TUE	WED	THR	FRI	SAT	TOTALS
A		117 $3,213.02	87 $3,256.07	91 $2,875.65	93 $3,483.26	91 $2,923.23	$0.00	479 $15,751.23
B		268 $8,599.58	224 $7,159.48	241 $7,642.51	217 $6,709.41	218 $6,928.22	11 $324.28	1179 $37,363.48
C		190 $5,373.53	261 $7,416.34	209 $5,973.88	216 $6,053.65	200 $6,018.80	6 $176.88	1082 $31,013.08
D		236 $6,971.43	207 $6,006.51	227 $6,669.74	218 $6,012.04	227 $6,604.08	20 $528.40	1135 $32,792.20
E		301 $8,901.32	209 $6,621.98	213 $5,869.41	229 $6,965.65	213 $6,189.19	9 $283.47	1174 $34,831.02
TOTAL HOSPITAL :		======== 1112 $33,058.88	======== 988 $30,460.38	======== 981 $29,031.19	======== 973 $29,224.01	======== 949 $28,663.52	======== 46 $1,313.03	======== 5049 $151,751.01

5/15/91 : 5/15/91

RUN TIME : 17.08.57

NATIONAL REHABILITATION HOSPITAL

OCCUPATIONAL THERAPY LOST TIME REPORT

FOR PERIOD ENDING   05/12/91
SUMMARY REPORT

NURSING STATION:

LOST TIME DESCRIPTION	MON	TUE	WED	THR	FRI	SAT	TOTALS
CANCEL-PATIENT				4			4
CANCEL THERAPY	14	21	28	13	8		84
CANCEL-TRANSPORT		2					2
LATE-NO SERVICE	2	4		2	4		12
NO SHOW	4	8	2	3	6		23
NO SHOW-SELF TRANSPORT			4				4
REFUSED SERVICE	4	5	6	10	5		30
SCHEDULE CONFLICT		4	4		4		12
SERVICE INTERRUPTED	2	4			1		7
SICK	2		2	1	2		7
TESTING	8	2	6	2	4		22
NURSE STATION TOTALS:	36	50	52	35	34		207

4/09/91 : 4/09/91
RUN TIME : 16.27.47

NATIONAL REHABILITATION HOSPITAL
OCCUPATION THERAPY PRODUCTIVITY REPORT

FOR PERIOD ENDING 03/31/91
MONTHLY SUMMARY REPORT

TEST DATA

TEAM		MON	TUE	WED	THR	FRI	SAT	TOTALS
A	TOTAL UNITS	215	220	209	196	239		1079
	REVENUE	$6,852.32	$8,357.06	$6,027.55	$7,151.70	$7,701.80	$0.00	$36,090.43
B	TOTAL UNITS	845	729	819	732	892	36	4053
	REVENUE	$26,322.76	$22,318.69	$26,486.42	$23,256.29	$28,704.40	$1,054.48	$128,143.04
C	TOTAL UNITS	857	819	891	879	938	113	4497
	REVENUE	$25,067.57	$23,412.80	$24,546.89	$25,004.33	$28,798.97	$2,896.04	$129,726.60
D	TOTAL UNITS	1055	985	946	1041	984	57	5068
	REVENUE	$30,410.85	$28,477.86	$28,188.76	$28,871.08	$29,749.62	$1,517.16	$147,215.33
E	TOTAL UNITS	1031	914	878	877	1129	45	4874
	REVENUE	$30,435.96	$26,733.32	$26,749.23	$26,572.82	$34,027.08	$1,272.20	$145,790.61
TOTAL HOSPITAL :		========	========	========	========	========	========	========
		4003	3667	3743	3725	4182	251	19571
		$119,089.46	$109,299.73	$111,998.85	$110,856.22	$128,981.87	$6,739.88	$586,966.01

6/08/91:   6/08/91
RUN TIME: 5.05.33

DEPT 210 OCCUPATIONAL THERAPY

NATIONAL REHABILITATION HOSPITAL
SERVICE DELIVERY EXCEPTION REPORTING
AS OF 6/08/91

(Reconciliation)

TEST DATA

THERAPIST	SCHEDULED SERVICE DATE	SCHEDULED TIME OF SERVICE	DOCUMENT CONTROL #	PATIENT NUMBER	PATIENT NAME
A	06/06/91	10:00	029	0000000	
	06/06/91	10:00	030	9104787	
	06/06/91	10:00	031	9103789	
	06/06/91	10:00	032	9104886	
	06/06/91	10:00	033	9103326	
	06/06/91	10:00	034	9101684	
	06/06/91	10:00	035	9101494	
B	06/06/91	01:00	131	9104134	
C	06/06/91	01:30	145	9105206	
	06/06/91	02:00	147	9105305	
D	06/06/91	11:00	169	9100793	
	06/06/91	11:00	170	9103458	
	06/06/91	11:00	171	9104142	
	06/06/91	11:00	172	9103755	
	06/06/91	11:00	173	9103821	
	06/06/91	11:00	174	9011453	
	06/06/91	12:00	175	9104142	
	06/06/91	12:00	176	9103755	
	06/06/91	12:00	177	9103797	
	06/06/91	12:00	178	9011453	
E	06/06/91	09:00	267	9101684	
	06/06/91	12:00	268	0000000	
F	06/06/91	02:00	297	9104761	

60B4

```
DATE 04/01/91  TIME 10:28 A.M.  PAGE   3  REPORT *SA2PM05

OT THERAPIST LOG. FOR PER. 03/26/91 TRUE 03/31/91
***
PT NO :
PT NO :
MED REC :
```

DATE OF SERVICE	. . .	DESCRIPTION OF SERVICE	THERAPIST NUMBER .	TOTAL QTY .	. .	SIGNATURE
03/27/91	21021381	OT-SM N/SENINT(1) *	24	1		
03/27/91	21021381	OT-SM N/SENINT(1)	24	1		
03/29/91	21021308	OT-SM NU/RGM(2-4)	26	3		
03/29/91	21022116	HOME MGMT (1)	28	2		
03/26/91	21021324	OT-SM NEU/COOR(1)	51	2		
03/26/91	21021449	OT-COGCON/COMP(1)	51	2		
03/27/91	21021282	OT-SM NUE/REF1(1)	51	4		
03/27/91	21021449	OT-COGCON/COMP(1)	51	2		
03/28/91	21021118	OT-REASS(1)	51	2		
03/28/91	21021282	OT-SM NUE/REF1(1)	51	2		
03/28/91	21022090	FUNCTIONAL MOBILITY (1)	51	2		
03/29/91	21021282	OT-SM NUE/REF1(1)	51	2		
03/29/91	21021449	OT-COGCON/COMP(1)	51	2		

* information in parenthesis indicates individual (1) or group (2-4) treatment

Consultant

10709 Colonial Woods Way
Louisville, KY 40223

Karen J. Miller, MOT, RMT, OTR/L
Consultant
(502) 244-0453

This is an example of a private practice that provides direct clinical services and specializes in program management consultancy to mental health settings and nursing homes. According to Ms. Miller, accurate records of productivity are essential to formulate bills. The Service Log (**Form A**) is used to document the consultants' activities, including actual time spent on such things as report writing, reviewing statistics, developing policies, etc. A copy is most often an office record only, but some facilities request a copy. Even services for which there is no charge are kept on this log.

The Bill for Service (**Form B**) is used to summarize the consultant's activities for the past billing period. It is designed to track and provide a record to the client of previous billing, payments received, and the current amount due. A copy is kept in the consultant's records as well as a standard accounting ledger for each client. This form is adaptable for hourly and flat-rate services. An additional signature line is provided for facilities that require a specific manager to approve contracted services before payment.

All forms in this section are courtesy of Karen J. Miller, MOT, RMT, OTR/L. Reprinted with permission.

SERVICE LOG
Service provided by: Karen J. Miller, MOT, RMT, OTR

Services to: _____

DATE	Time IN	Time OUT	Total Hours	Services

KAREN J. MILLER, MOT, RMT, LOTR
Occupational Therapist
Music Therapist

BILL FOR SERVICE

TO: DATE:

Billing Period: _____ to _____

Billing Rate: _____ per _____

DATE	SERVICE	HOURS	TOTAL

Previous Balance	– Payments	+ Current Balance	= Balance Due

Make Check Payable To:

Karen J. Miller
10709 Colonial Woods Way
Louisville, KY 40223

Signed: _____
        Karen J. Miller

Services Approved by:

_____

                                    Date

Northwestern Memorial Hospital

303 East Superior Street
Chicago, IL 60611

Letty Sargant, MS, OTR/L
Director, Rehabilitation Services
(312) 908-2526

Type of setting:
General Hospital

Number of beds:
720

Total number of FTEs for this setting:
13

Productivity standard (in hours per day):
OTR Entry Level: 5.2 hrs.
OTR Inter. Level: 5.2-5.6 hrs.
OTR Adv. Level: 5.2-5.6 hrs.
COTA Entry Level: 5.2 hrs.
COTA Inter. Level: 5.2-5.6 hrs.
COTA Adv. Level: 5.2-5.6 hrs.
Manager/Director: 0 hrs.
Fieldwork Supervisor/Coordinator: 4 hrs.
Clinical Specialist: 5.2-5.6 hrs.

Two measures of productivity are used on an ongoing basis. One monitors the productivity of individual therapists; the second monitors the overall department productivity.

Individual staff productivity is determined by calculating each therapist's direct billable time (DBT). Daily patient treatments/procedures are documented on the Occupational Therapy Clinical Service Log (**Form A**). The relative value units (RVUs) designated for each procedure are totalled and entered on **Form B**, the Professional Activity Summary. All direct patient care activities and documentation time are included in the time-based procedure charges.

At the end of each week, the therapists total their weekly DBT and submit Form B to their supervisor. The Professional Activity Summary indicates absences, caseload, and missed treatments. In addition, therapists' nonbillable time (NBT), such as meetings, rounds, and student supervision, is identified. Data from Form B are summarized by the supervisor and transferred to **Form C**, the Supervisor's Weekly Summary. This is used to evaluate productivity trends of individual staff and service areas. Missed treatments are monitored to identify staffing issues and needs.

Department productivity is calculated and reported via the Management Engineering Department. Two biweekly productivity reports (**Attachments A and B**) are generated by Management Engineering through employee time cards and the computerized charge (procedure) entry system. Attachment A details total staff productive hours, nonproductive hours, and total hours. These hours are compared to RVUs of total procedures charged. A standard for hours per RVUs is determined by the director during the annual operating budget process.

Attachment A also compares the fixed and variable FTEs to volume (RVUs) to determine a flexible budget variance. This calculation identifies overstaffing or understaffing, and is used to justify additional FTEs.

Attachment B is a graphic representation of the following data that are identified in Attachment A: (1) paid hours, (2) paid hours per RVU, (3) RVUs, and (4) productive hours per RVU. The report allows the

Continues on next page

visualization of actual data as they compare to budget—90% of budget and 110% of budget.

Inpatient and outpatient procedures and referrals are logged onto **Forms D** and **E**. Form D details referrals from specific service areas and hospital buildings. It also identifies new referrals and carryover of referrals from the previous month. Form D is used for monthly analysis of referral service trends. Form E (Monthly Analysis of Service) compares month-to-month volume changes in ambulatory care and inpatient services.

Annual department productivity is entered on **Attachment C**. Average procedures per month are compared to total FTE ratio. Also, average new referrals and caseload per month are tracked to create a historical record of occupational therapy department statistics.

All forms and attachments in this section are courtesy of Northwestern Memorial Hospital, Chicago, IL. Reprinted with permission.

Northwestern Memorial Hospital
OCCUPATIONAL THERAPY CLINICAL SERVICE LOG

PAV/RM.NO. _____

PATIENT NAME _____ ACCT. NO. _____ PRIMARY THERAPIST _____

DATE REFERRAL RECEIVED _____ MED. REC. NO. _____ PHYSCIAN

DATE	GEN	10	15	30	45	60	INIT	SUPPLIES-407	SUPPLY COST	TOTAL TIME	DONE

FORM NO. 501052   TOTAL TREATMENTS _____   TOTAL TIME--->

REFERRAL CODES

10				
001				General

15	30	45	60	
	987	995		Initial Assessment
33316	33993	32920	32938	Developmental Evaluation
555	563	571	589	General Evaluation
	080		090	Hand Evaluations
105	110	120	130	Hand Rehabilitation
33324	32946	32953	32961	Developmental Treatment

15	30	45	60	
712	720	738	746	Independent Daily Living Tr.I
795	803	811	829	Neuromuscular Integration Tr
837	845	852	860	Neuromuscular Inegration Tr.
878	886	894	902	Sensory/Cog. Integration Tr. I
140	150	160	170	Hand Rehab. Adj.
951	969	977	985	Orthotic fabrication
019	027	035	043	Equipment fabrication
	33994			Dressing Change

LYMPHADENMA

30	60	
33999	34000	Edema Evaluation
34001	34002	Manual Therapy
	33998	Compression Therapy

FORM NO. 501052

NORTHWESTERN MEMORIAL HOSPITAL
DEPARTMENT OF REHABILITATION SERVICES

PROFESSIONAL ACTIVITY SUMMARY

EMPLOYEE #:_____ STAFF/STUDENT NAME:_____

_____Supervisor_____Staff_____Temporary Staff_____Student

Service
Assignment:_____Ortho_____Neuro/Neuro Sx_____Med/Sx_____Ped

WEEK:_____to_____

	MON	TUES	WED	THURS	FRI	SAT	WEEKLY TOTAL
HOURS WORKED							
HOURS OFF and CODE							
DBT (in minutes)							
NBT							
STUDENT TRAINING							
MEETINGS							
CONTINUING EDUCATION							
OTHER							
CASELOAD							
PTS NOT SEEN							
PTS SHOULD HAVE TX							

CODES FOR HOURS OFF (Same as Time Card Codes)

COMP = Department Comp. Time
CE   = Continuing Education (8 hour programs only)
S = Sick V = Vacation   H/FH = Holiday/Floating Holiday
JD = Jury Duty WC = Workmen's Comp. DF = Death in Family

prof-act.sum

SUPERVISOR'S WEEKLY SUMMARY
PRODUCTIVITY STATISTICS

Week of	5/13	5/20	5/27	6/3	6/10	6/17	6/24	7/1	7/15	7/22	7/29	8/5
Mary												
Prod %												
Avg daily csld												
Total missed Rx												
Frank												
Prod %												
Avg daily csld												
Total missed Rx												
Paula												
Prod %												
Avg daily csld												
Total missed Rx												
Margaret												
Prod %												
Avg daily csld												
Total missed Rx												
Student												
Prod %												
Avg daily csld												
Total missed Rx												
00												
Prod %												
Avg daily csld												
Total missed Rx												

NORTHWESTERN MEMORIAL HOSPITAL
DEPARTMENT OF REHABILITATION SERVICES

Division _____ (562 OT) _____ (563 PT)

Activity Summary for _____ (Mo) _____ (Yr)

Caseload

Previous month carry over
Inpatient _____
Outpatient _____
Total _____

New referrals for month
Inpatient _____
Outpatient _____
Total _____

Total referrals
Inpatient _____
Outpatient _____
Total _____

Visits and Procedures

Inpatient visits _____
Outpatient visits _____
Total _____

Inpatient procedures _____
Outpatient procedures _____
Total _____

New Referrals: Patient Location

Wesley [1] _____
Passavant [2] _____
Prentice [3] _____
Psych. [4] _____
Olson [5] _____

New referral service origin for month (Inpatients)

_____ Anes [1]	_____ Comm Med [6]	_____ Optha [11]	_____ Phys Med [16]	_____ Cardio [22]
_____ Comm Hea [2]	_____ Renal [7]	_____ Ortho [12]	_____ Psych [17]	_____ Surg [23]
_____ Derm [3]	_____ Neuro [8]	_____ Otolar [13]	_____ Radiol [17]	_____ Plast [23]
_____ Dent [4]	_____ Gyne [9]	_____ Path [14]	_____ Gen Surg [18]	_____ Urol [24]
_____ Med [5]	_____ Obst [10]	_____ Peds [15]	_____ Neuro Surg [19]	_____ Hand [25]
			_____ [20]	_____ Other [26]

New referral service origin for month (Outpatients)

_____ Anes [1]	_____ Comm Med [6]	_____ Optha [11]	_____ Phys Med [16]	_____ Cardio [22]
_____ Comm Hea [2]	_____ Renal [7]	_____ Ortho [12]	_____ Psych [17]	_____ Surg [23]
_____ Derm [3]	_____ Neuro [8]	_____ Otolar [13]	_____ Radiol [17]	_____ Plast [23]
_____ Dent [4]	_____ Gyne [9]	_____ Path [14]	_____ Gen Surg [18]	_____ Urol [24]
_____ Med [5]	_____ Obst [10]	_____ Peds [15]	_____ Neuro Surg [19]	_____ Hand [25]
			_____ [20]	_____ Other [26]

Northwestern Memorial Hospital
Department of Rehabilitation Services

MONTHLY ANALYSIS OF SERVICE

Fiscal Year _____

	AMBULATORY CARE SERVICES (OUTPATIENTS)		INPATIENT SERVICES	
	Patients	Procedures	Patients	Procedures
September				
October				
November				
December				
January				
February				
March				
April				
May				
June				
July				
August				
TOTAL				

PAGE 107
21-FEB-91 09:06 AM
PROFLEX.RPH
ERE16.DBH

PRINT DATE:
CONTROL FILE:
DATA BASE:

NORTHWESTERN MEMORIAL HOSPITAL
FLEX HOURS AND HOURS PER RVU BY PAY PERIOD
FOR THE PAY PERIOD ENDING 2-16-91

07301050 REHABILITAT: 562 OCCUPATIONAL THE

	PERIOD 1 ENDING 9-1-90	PERIOD 2 ENDING 9-15-90	PERIOD 3 ENDING 9-29-90	PERIOD 4 ENDING 10-13-90	PERIOD 5 ENDING 10-27-90	PERIOD 6 ENDING 11-10-90	PERIOD 7 ENDING 11-24-90	PERIOD 8 ENDING 12-8-90	PERIOD 9 ENDING 12-22-90	PERIOD 10 ENDING 1-5-91	PERIOD 11 ENDING 1-19-91	PERIOD 12 ENDING 2-2-91	PERIOD 13 ENDING 2-16-91	YTD
REGULAR HOURS	939	653	759	825	774	949	702	891	830	572	876	897	929	10596
OVERTIME HOURS	0	0	0	0	0	0	0	4	0	0	0	0	0	4
AGENCY HOURS	0	0	0	111	0	160	143	92	80	16	80	0	0	682
PRODUCTIVE HOURS	939	653	759	936	774	1109	845	987	910	588	956	897	929	11282
VACATION HOURS	52	136	100	20	0	127	96	49	32	148	0	80	24	864
SICK HOURS	16	6	36	41	6	8	8	34	12	24	44	16	17	268
HOLIDAY HOURS	8	88	8	0	0	24	93	16	35	186	0	4	0	462
OTHER HOURS	0	0	0	0	24	0	0	8	0	0	0	0	0	32
UNPRODUCTIVE HOURS	76	230	144	61	30	159	197	107	79	358	44	100	41	1626
TOTAL PAID HOURS	1015	883	903	997	804	1268	1042	1094	989	946	1000	997	970	12908
BENEFIT %	7.5	26.0	15.9	6.9	3.7	14.4	21.9	10.7	8.7	38.5	4.8	10.0	4.2	13.3
TOTAL PAID FTES	12.7	11.0	11.3	12.5	10.1	15.9	13.0	13.7	12.4	11.8	12.5	12.5	12.1	12.4
ANNUAL BUDGET FTES	12.8	12.8	12.8	12.8	12.8	12.8	12.8	12.8	12.8	12.8	12.8	12.8	12.8	12.8
VARIANCE	.1	1.8	1.5	.3	2.7	-3.1	-.2	-.9	.4	1.0	.3	.3	.7	.4
PROD HRS/100 RVUS	4.03	3.19	4.00	4.66	3.45	4.37	3.79	4.15	3.73	3.83	3.94	4.12	4.66	3.99
UNPROD HRS/100 RVUS	.33	1.12	.76	.30	.13	.63	.88	.45	.32	2.33	.18	.46	.21	.58
TOTAL HRS/100 RVUS	4.36	4.31	4.76	4.96	3.58	5.00	4.67	4.60	4.05	6.16	4.12	4.58	4.87	4.57
BUDGET HRS/100 RVUS	4.79	4.79	4.79	4.79	4.79	4.79	4.79	4.79	4.79	4.79	4.79	4.79	4.79	4.79
VARIANCE	.43	.48	.03	-.17	1.21	-.21	.12	.19	.74	-1.37	.67	.21	-.08	.22
CURRENT PROCEDURES	797	661	661	633	750	917	780	755	736	546	876	767	663	9542
ACCRUAL	0	2	14	4	-1	37	12	3	102	80	6	1	6	266
LATE CHARGE ADJ	2	12	-10	-5	38	-25	-9	99	-22	-74	-5	5	0	6
TOTAL PROCEDURES	799	675	665	632	787	929	783	857	816	552	877	773	669	9814
RVUS	23285	20500	18955	20101	22434	25389	22278	23767	24427	15365	24278	21760	19924	282463
RVUS/PROC	29.14	30.37	28.50	31.81	28.51	27.33	28.45	27.73	29.94	27.84	27.68	28.15	29.78	28.78

	PERIOD 1 ENDING 9-1-90	PERIOD 2 ENDING 9-15-90	PERIOD 3 ENDING 9-29-90	PERIOD 4 ENDING 10-13-90	PERIOD 5 ENDING 10-27-90	PERIOD 6 ENDING 11-10-90	PERIOD 7 ENDING 11-24-90	PERIOD 8 ENDING 12-8-90	PERIOD 9 ENDING 12-22-90	PERIOD 10 ENDING 1-5-91	PERIOD 11 ENDING 1-19-91	PERIOD 12 ENDING 2-2-91	PERIOD 13 ENDING 2-16-91	YTD
FLEX BUDGET ANALYSIS														
FIXED HOURS	336	336	336	336	336	336	336	336	336	336	336	336	336	4368
VARIABLE HOURS	749	659	610	646	721	816	716	764	786	494	781	700	641	8083
TOTAL FLEX HOURS	1085	995	946	982	1057	1152	1052	1100	1122	830	1117	1036	977	13451
FIXED BUDGET FTES	4.2	4.2	4.2	4.2	4.2	4.2	4.2	4.2	4.2	4.2	4.2	4.2	4.2	4.2
VARIABLE BUDGET FTE	9.4	8.2	7.6	8.1	9.0	10.2	9.0	9.6	9.8	6.2	9.8	8.8	8.0	8.7
TOTAL BUDGET FEES	13.6	12.4	11.8	12.3	13.2	14.4	13.2	13.8	14.0	10.4	14.0	13.0	12.2	12.9
FLEX BUD VARIANCE	.9	1.4	.5	-.2	3.1	-1.5	.2	.1	1.6	-1.4	1.5	.5	.1	.5
FLEX BUD HR/100 RVU	4.66	4.85	4.99	4.89	4.71	4.54	4.72	4.63	4.59	5.40	4.60	4.76	4.90	4.76
FLEX HR RVU VAR	.30	.54	.23	-.07	1.13	-.46	.05	.03	.54	-.76	.48	.18	.03	.19

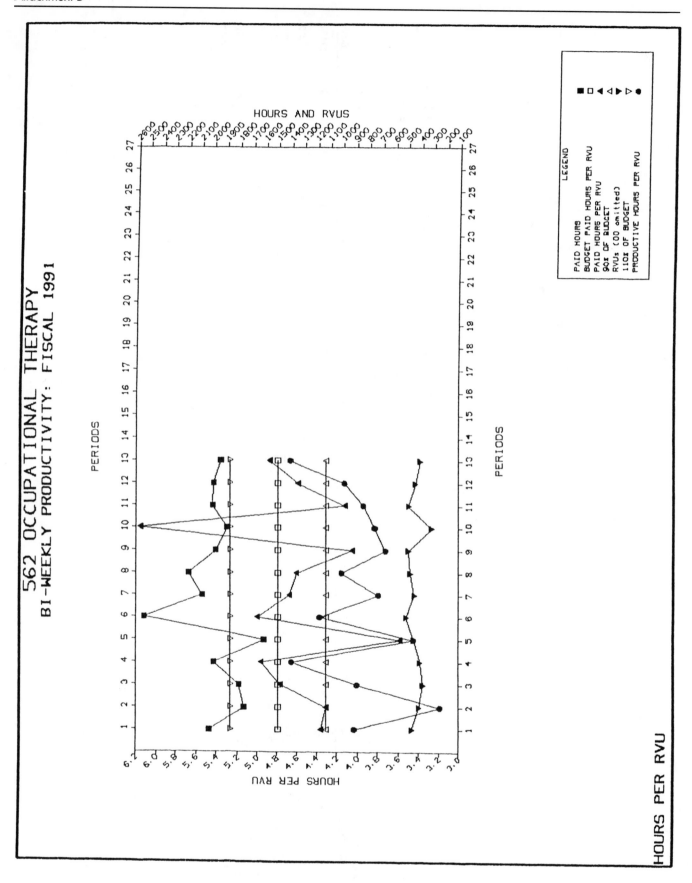

562 OCCUPATIONAL THERAPY
BI-WEEKLY PRODUCTIVITY: FISCAL 1991

LEGEND

PAID HOURS
BUDGET PAID HOURS PER RVU
PAID HOURS PER RVU
90% OF BUDGET
RVUs (00 omitted)
110% OF BUDGET
PRODUCTIVE HOURS PER RVU

HOURS AND RVUS

HOURS PER RVU

PERIODS

HOURS PER RVU

NORTHWESTERN MEMORIAL HOSPITAL
OCCUPATIONAL THERAPY DEPARTMENT STATISTICS

FISCAL YEARS 1984-1990

	1984	1985	1986	1987	1988	1989	1990
Total Number Patient Treatments/Year							
Inpatients	12,018	10,226	9,606	9,393	9,959	10,573	10,828
Outpatients	2,525	4,500	4,922	6,410	6,972	5,344	4,034
Total No. of Treatments	14,572	14,726	14,528	15,803	16,931	15,917	14,862
Average/Month	1,214	1,227	1,211	1,317	1,411	1,326	1,239
Average Procedures/Mo/FTE	106	109	102	102	109	104	95
Total Number New Patient Referrals per Year (1)							
Inpatient	1,736	1,651	1,761	2,044	2,150	2,365	2,396
Outpatient	213	228	281	468	479	432	379
Total New Referrals	1,949	1,879	2,042	2,512	2,629	2,787	2,775
Average per Month	162	157	170	209	219	232	231
Average Caseload Per Mo. (2) (old and new patients)	271	331	404	506	513	491	552
Professional & Support Staff	11.4	11.3	11.9	12.9	13.0	12.7	13.0
	FTE's	FTE's	FTE's	FTE's	FTE's	FTE's	FTE's
OTR's	7	7.6	8.0	8.0	8.0	8.7	9.0
COTA's	2.4	1.7	1.9	2.9	3.0	2.0	2.0
Support	2.0	2.0	2.0	2.0	2.0	2.0	2.0

(1) Patients are classified as new when a treatment request is received. For each subsequent readmission to the hospital and new O.T. treatment request the same fiscal year, the patient is classified as new.

(2) Patients are classified as old when they are carried over from month to month on our treatment program. The average caseload per month included both in- and outpatients and old and new patients.

Professional Rehabilitation Center, Inc.

12825 Flushing Meadows Drive
St. Louis, MO 63131

Sheryl K. Schwartz, OTR
Director of Occupational Therapy
(314) 821-0008

This rehabilitation agency provides geriatric services throughout metropolitan St. Louis and provides direct billing for all rehabilitation services.

The occupational therapy department has 16 FTEs, including a director. Productivity standards for full-time, salaried staff are based on an average of six patients per day at a minimum of 24 billable units per day (15-minute units). **Form A** is used by the director and area coordinator of the occupational therapy department to track productivity and help plan for proper staffing and patient coverage. Information for Form A is obtained every Friday from each therapist, who reports visits/units completed for that week as well as projected number of visits for the following week. **Form B** is an agency form completed and turned in at the end of each month. Therapists from every discipline at each facility complete this form. Billing information is taken directly from Form B. **Form C** is for the department director and is generated by the finance department. This form highlights necessary revenue and unit expectations based on monthly salary. Finally, **Forms D** and **E** are monthly and quarterly productivity reports used by the director and generated by the finance department. For this agency, meeting your productivity goal is ranked as 1/3 of the annual performance criteria for bonuses, with 1/3 allotted to provision of a quality product, and 1/3 allotted to a pleasant working environment.

All forms in this section are courtesy of Professional Rehabilitation Center, Inc., St. Louis, MO. Reprinted with permission.

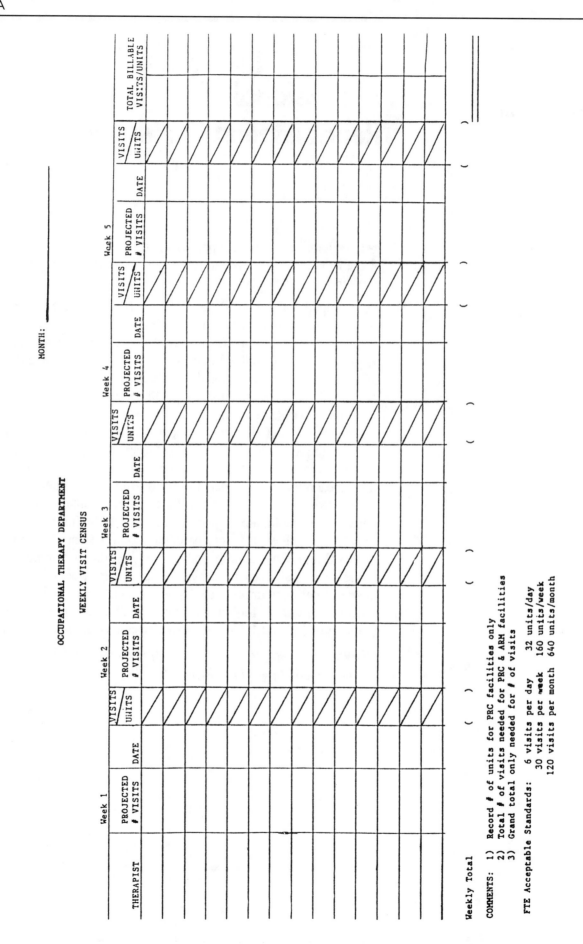

OCCUPATIONAL THERAPY DEPARTMENT

WEEKLY VISIT CENSUS

MONTH:

THERAPIST	Week 1			Week 2			Week 3			Week 4			Week 5			TOTAL BILLABLE VISITS/UNITS
	PROJECTED # VISITS	DATE	VISITS/UNITS	PROJECTED # VISITS	DATE	VISITS/UNITS	PROJECTED # VISITS	DATE	VISITS/UNITS	PROJECTED # VISITS	DATE	VISITS/UNITS	PROJECTED # VISITS	DATE	VISITS/UNITS	

Weekly Total

COMMENTS:
1) Record # of units for PRC facilities only
2) Total # of visits needed for PRC & ARM facilities
3) Grand total only needed for # of visits

FTE Acceptable Standards:
6 visits per day   32 units/day
30 visits per week   160 units/week
120 visits per month   640 units/month

PATIENT VISIT RECORD

PERIOD ENDING: Oct. 31, 1991

EMPLOYEE NAME: Sheryl Schwartz, OTR   Rest Easy Nursing Home

E - EVALUATION
D/C - DISCHARGE
CV - CANCELED VISIT
CC - CONSULTATION
R - REFUSED
H - HOLD

PATIENT NAME (Last, First)	1	2	3	4	5	6	7	8	9	10	11	12	13	14	15	16	17	18	19	20	21	22	23	24	25	26	27	28	29	30	31	Total Visits	Total Units	Comments
Jones, Mary 5x/wk				SS			SS	SS	SS	SS	SS			SS	SS	SS	SS	SS			SS	SS	SS		SS			SS	SS	SS	SS	17	82	↓ to 3x/wk 10/21/91
Earl, Thomas 3x/wk		SS	SS	SS			①	SS	②	SS	SS			SS	SS	SS	SS	SS			SS	SS	SS		DC 10/23/91							9	45	DC to home
Good, Johnny 5x/wk		SS	SS	SS			SS	SS	SS	SS	SS			SS	SS	SS	SS	SS			SS	SS	SS	Ⓡ	Ⓡ			SS	SS	SS	SS	20	95	
Snail, Irma 3x/wk							E SS		SS		SS			SS		SS		SS		DC 10/17/91												6	32	@ hand splint 10/11

TOTAL

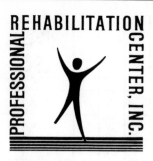

ELLEN A. FRIESEN, PRESIDENT

(314) 821-0008

OCCUPATIONAL THERAPY DEPARTMENT
PRODUCTIVITY GOALS

Employee	Monthly Salary	Revenue Goal	Unit Goal

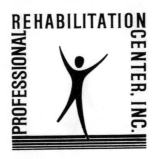

ELLEN A. FRIESEN, PRESIDENT   (314) 821-0008

OCCUPATIONAL THERAPY
PRODUCTIVITY SUMMARY
July 1991

Total Treatments

Treatments By Employed Staff

Treatments By Contractors

****

ANALYSIS OF PRODUCTIVY OF EMPLOYED STAFF

Treatments

Treatment Days Worked

Treatments Per Treatment Day

Average Time Per Treatment
(In Minutes)

Professional Rehabilitation Center, Inc.   133

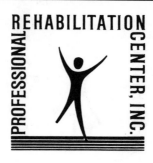

ELLEN A. FRIESEN, PRESIDENT   (314) 821-0008

SAMPLE FORM

DEPARTMENT OF OCCUPATIONAL THERAPY
PRODUCTIVITY ANALYSIS

THERAPIST	ARM TX'S	PRC TX'S	TOTAL TX'S	DAYS WORKED	TX'S PER DAY	RATIO REV:SAL
Jones, M., OTR	0	102	102	21	4.9	4.3
Hill, A., COTA	77	7	84	20	4.2	2.7
Smith, T., OTR	15	112	127	21.50	5.9	3.8
Williams, W., COTA	42	43	85	17.50	4.9	3.0
Yount, C., OTR	83	14	97	22	4.4	2.4
	217	278	495	102	4.86	3.24

CONTRACT STAFF

King, Carol, OTR	23	18				

TOTALS	240	296				

South Carolina Division of Home Health Services

South Carolina Department of Health
and Environmental Control
Division of Home Health Services
2600 Bull Street
Columbia, SC 29201

Tina Scott, OTR/L
Occupational Therapy Consultant
(803) 737-3957

This is an example of a state home health system that includes 15 separate home health agencies under one administrative regime. They do not have productivity and FTEs for each agency calculated separately, but do strive for a state average of 5.25 visits per day for both OTRs and COTAs. They have only exempt, part-time, and contract therapists, no FTEs. Therapists are paid only for visits made, with the exception of a few administrative hours per month paid on a half-visit basis. Because they provide services for every county in the state, there is a chronic shortage of therapists and always more visits possible than actually made. Therefore, although FTEs and productivity are calculated for each discipline, they do not carry much weight for the therapy services.

The therapist records time on the bottom portion of the Clinical Note Form (**Form A**). The information is then transferred to the Home Health Services Report, which is the patient billing form (**Form B**). The therapist also completes the Monthly Expense Report (**Form C**) and the Time and Activity Report (not shown). Data from the latter are part of the computerized Personnel Cost Accountability System, which results in reports like **Attachment A**.

All forms and attachments in this section are courtesy of the South Carolina Department of Health and Environmental Control, Columbia, SC. Reprinted with permission.

SOUTH CAROLINA DEPARTMENT OF HEALTH AND ENVIRONMENTAL CONTROL
DIVISION OF HOME HEALTH SERVICES

CLINICAL NOTES

TREATMENT PLAN	DATE:	DATE:	DATE:	DATE:

COORDINATION/
COMMUNICATION

SIGNATURE AND TITLE

VISIT DATE	CASE STATUS	PERSONNEL NUMBER		TRAVEL		TOTAL MILES	TIME IN MINUTES			SUPPLIES		
				TIME	ODOM		HOME	OFFICE	TRAVEL	TYPE	AMOUNT	CODE
			D									
			A									
			D									
			A									
			D									
			A									
			D									
			A									

CASE STATUS KEY: 1. Admission   2. Readmission   3. New by Transfer
4. Evaluation   5. Reevaluation   6. Discharge
7. Supervision 8. Dual   9. No Visit 0. Revisit

PATIENT ID# _____

PATIENT NAME _____
                    LAST   FIRST   MI

_____
                DISCIPLINE

DHEC 1639 (4/88)

DATE OF BIRTH _____

Managing Productivity in Occupational Therapy

SOUTH CAROLINA DEPARTMENT OF HEALTH AND ENVIRONMENTAL CONTROL
DIVISION OF HOME HEALTH SERVICES

Clinical Notes (Flow Slip)
(Instructions for Completing)

PURPOSE:

The flow slip provides for, each home visit, systematic documentation
of (1) billing information and (2) therapy or social work plans and
interventions and patient's response.   One, two, three or four visits
may be entered on each flow slip.

EXPLANATIONS AND DEFINITIONS Item-by-Item Instructions)

Treatment Plans: List treatment plans or interventions in the first
column.

Visit Columns: Enter date of each visit at the top of the column. In
boxes corresponding to the treatment plans, enter appropriate
information regarding service given. In the boxes corresponding to
coordination/communications, enter conferences and contacts made to
agency personnel, physicians, community resources or patient/family
regarding the patient's care.

Signature: For each visit, enter legal signature and title of
individual providing service.

Billing Information: Following each visit, complete date of the visit,
case status (see key), personnel number, home, office and travel times,
mileage, supplies issued to the patient and discipline.

Identifying Information: Enter patient's identification number, name
and date of birth.

OFFICE MECHANICS AND FILING: The therapist or social worker submits
the flow slip to the agency weekly. The clerk transfers billing
information to appropriate form. The original clinical documentation
is filed in the patient's clinical record and retained according to
agency policy. The carbon copy is retained by the therapist or social
worker.

DHEC 1639 (4/88)

SOUTH CAROLINA DEPARTMENT OF HEALTH AND ENVIRONMENTAL CONTROL
HOME HEALTH SERVICES REPORT

(01) _ — Patient's Last Name

(02) _ — Patient's First Name and Initial

(03) _ — Street Address

(04) _ — City, State, Zip Code

(05) _ _ _ _ _	Patient Number	
(06) _ _ _ _ _ _	Episode Date	

(07) _ _ _ _ _ _ _ _ _ _ _ _ _   HIC Number
(08) _ _ _ _ _ _ _ _ _ _ _ _   MID Number
(09) _ _ _ _ _ _ _ _ _ _ _   Other Coverage Number
(10) _ _ _ _ _ _ _ _ _   Birth Date (MMDDYYYY)
(11) _ _ _ _ _ _   Date Plan Established
(12) _ _ _ _ _   Physician's License

(13) _ _ _ • _ _ _   Primary Diagnosis Code
(14) _ _ _ • _ _ _   Secondary Diagnosis (1)
(15) _ _ _ • _ _ _   Secondary Diagnosis (2)
(16) _ _ _ • _ _ _   Secondary Diagnosis (3)

(17) _ _ _ _ • _ _   Discount Amount
(18) _ _ _ _ • _ _   Amount Received Other
(19) _ _ _   Payment Sources (A)
(20) _   Portion of Charges Billed (B)

(22) _ _   County Code (C)
(23) _   Billing: 1-Medicare 2-Medicaid
(24) _   Other Billing

(25) —   Form Status (D)

(26) _   Sex (E)
(27) _   Employment Related: A-Yes B-No

(28) _ _   Reason Not Admitted (F)
(29) _ _   Source of Referral (G)
(30) _ _   School Years Completed
(31) _ _   Number Problems Identified
(32) _ _   Number Problems Resolved
(33) _   Functional Level at Discharge (H)
(34) _   Reason Discharged (I)

(35) _   Number of Interrupted Services
(36) _   Living Arrangements (J)
(37) _   Functional Level at Admission (H)
(38) _   Level of Care (K)
(39) _   Race (L)

(21) CHARGES

Supplies	Appliances	Payor (A)
$ _ _ _ • _ _	$ _ _ _ • _ _	_
$ _ _ _ • _ _	$ _ _ _ • _ _	_

Appliances:

Supplies:

Contract Services:

Other Insurance:

(40) Visit Date	Case Status	Personnel No.	TIME IN MINUTES			Modi-fier	Payor (A)
			Home	Office	Travel		
_ _ _ _ _	_	_ _ _ _ _	_ _ _	_ _ _	_ _ _	_ _ _	_
_ _ _ _ _	_	_ _ _ _ _	_ _ _	_ _ _	_ _ _	_ _ _	_
_ _ _ _ _	_	_ _ _ _ _	_ _ _	_ _ _	_ _ _	_ _ _	_
_ _ _ _ _	_	_ _ _ _ _	_ _ _	_ _ _	_ _ _	_ _ _	_
_ _ _ _ _	_	_ _ _ _ _	_ _ _	_ _ _	_ _ _	_ _ _	_
_ _ _ _ _	_	_ _ _ _ _	_ _ _	_ _ _	_ _ _	_ _ _	_
_ _ _ _ _	_	_ _ _ _ _	_ _ _	_ _ _	_ _ _	_ _ _	_
_ _ _ _ _	_	_ _ _ _ _	_ _ _	_ _ _	_ _ _	_ _ _	_
_ _ _ _ _	_	_ _ _ _ _	_ _ _	_ _ _	_ _ _	_ _ _	_
_ _ _ _ _	_	_ _ _ _ _	_ _ _	_ _ _	_ _ _	_ _ _	_
_ _ _ _ _	_	_ _ _ _ _	_ _ _	_ _ _	_ _ _	_ _ _	_
_ _ _ _ _	_	_ _ _ _ _	_ _ _	_ _ _	_ _ _	_ _ _	_
_ _ _ _ _	_	_ _ _ _ _	_ _ _	_ _ _	_ _ _	_ _ _	_
_ _ _ _ _	_	_ _ _ _ _	_ _ _	_ _ _	_ _ _	_ _ _	_
_ _ _ _ _	_	_ _ _ _ _	_ _ _	_ _ _	_ _ _	_ _ _	_
_ _ _ _ _	_	_ _ _ _ _	_ _ _	_ _ _	_ _ _	_ _ _	_
_ _ _ _ _	_	_ _ _ _ _	_ _ _	_ _ _	_ _ _	_ _ _	_
_ _ _ _ _	_	_ _ _ _ _	_ _ _	_ _ _	_ _ _	_ _ _	_

Case Status: 1=Admission 2=Readmission 3=New By Transfer 4=Evaluation 5=Reassessment
6=Discharge 7=Supervision 8=Dual 9=No Visit 0=Revisit

PRIVATE INSURANCE COMPANIES

NAME _____

ADDRESS _____

NAME _____

ADDRESS _____

CODE TABLES

Code Table A
Payment Source
Payor Code

A.	Medicare A	H.	
B.	Medicare B	I.	Self
C.	Medicaid	J.	Other
D.	VA	K.	Hospice
E.	Champus	L.	1483 Billing
F.	Other	M.	Denied Medicare
G.	Community Agency	N.	Denied Medicaid

Code Table B
Portion of Charges to be Billed

1.	None	4.	75%
2.	25%	5.	Full
3.	50%		

Code Table D
Form Status

1.	Evaluation	6.	Continued Service
3.	New	7.	Data Change
4.	Discharge	9.	Adjustment
5.	New-Discharge		

Code Table E
Sex

1.	Male	2.	Female
M.	Male	F.	Female

Code Table G
Source of Referral

1.	Self/Related	6.	Other Agency Non-DHEC
2.	Individual, Non Related	7.	Out-Patient Department
3.	Doctors	8.	Nursing Home
4.	Hospital	9.	VA
5.	Other Division, DHEC	10.	News Media
		11.	Other
		12.	Community Long Term Care

Code Table H
Functional Level

1. None
2. Needs Assistance in Household Activities.
3. Needs Minimal Assistance
4. Needs Moderate Assistance
5. Dependent for Personal Care
6. Died

Code Table I
Reason Discharged

1. Therapeutic Goals Met
2. Therapeutic Goals Not Attainable
3. Admitted to Hospital
4. Admitted to Skilled Nursing Facility
5. Died
6. Transferred
7. Moved
8. No longer meets criteria for home care
9. Other

Code Table J
Living Arrangements

1. Alone
2. Alone with Outside Help
3. With Family
4. Alone with Homemaker
5. With Friends
6. Twenty-four Hour Companion
7. Other

Code Table K
Level of Care

1. Concentrated (Intensive)
2. Intermediate
3. Basic
4. Terminal

Code Table L
Race

1.	White	2.	All Others

MONTHLY TRAVEL EXPENSE REPORT

SOUTH CAROLINA DEPARTMENT OF HEALTH AND ENVIRONMENTAL CONTROL

SSN: _____

Name:
Street:
City & State:
Zip:

Date:
Official Hdqts. City:
City of Residence:
Cost Center Title:

☐ Check Block for Travel Expenses Paid to Non-State Employee and Explain Purpose Below.

DATE MO DA	D A	TIME	AM PM	DESTINATION OF TRAVEL FROM	TO		IN STATE	OUT OF STATE	50504 / 50514 Auto Miles	50901 Per Diem	50501 / 50511 Meals	50502 / 50512 Lodging	50503 / 50513 Air Trans	50505 / 50515 Other Trans	50506 / 50516 Misc. Travel Expense	52350 Registration Fees
						1			50504	50901	50501	50502	50503	50505	50506	52350
						2		1 or 2	50514 × ___	50901 ___	50511	50512	50513	50515	50516	52350

Total 1 — 50504, 50901, 50501, 50502, 50503, 50505, 50506, 52350
Total 2 — 50514, 50901, 50511, 50512, 50513, 50515, 50516, 52350

Grand Total

Travel Advance (50580) $ _____

I hereby certify or affirm that the above expenses were actually incurred by me as necessary traveling expenses in the performance of my official duties; any meals or lodging included in a conference or convention registration fee paid by the Agency have been deducted from this travel claim; and that this claim is true and correct in every material matter and conforms with the requirements of State laws, rules and regulations.

SIGNATURE _____ Date _____
APPROVED _____ Date _____
Date _____

	1-2	3-5	6-10	11	18-22	39-43	45-52
KF	T Code	Voucher No.	P	Vendor No.	Manual Vouch	Amount
P 2	615		1			

T Code	P	Cost Center	Fund	Class	Analytical	Amount
3-5	11	12-16	17-20	21-25	26-35	52-59
	2					
	2					
	2					
	2					

T Code	P	Cost Center	Fund	Class	Analytical	Amount
	2					
	2					
	2					
	2					
	2					
	2					
	2					

DHEC 103 - Page 1 (Rev. 5/84)

STATE TOTALS — 1ST QTR

	JULY 88	AUGUST 88	SEPT 88	TOTALS 1ST QTR	TARGET 1ST QTR	% TARGET MET	MBO PROJECTED F.T.E.	F.T.E. 1ST QTR	1ST QTR AVG VISITS PER DAY
RN VISITS	18385	19382	18925	56692	58065	98%	267.73	231.97	4.72
LPN VISITS	684	644	540	1868	2380	78%	8.80	7.50	4.82
ALL NURSE VISITS	19069	20026	19465	58560	60445	97%	276.53	239.46	4.73
HSW VISITS	1115	1197	1007	3319	3922	85%	19.52	15.29	4.19
PT VISITS	4211	4484	4154	12849	10726	120%	42.44	35.99	6.90
ST VISITS	573	659	616	1848	2173	85%	9.20	5.06	7.06
OT VISITS	646	814	685	2145	2084	103%	9.17	7.48	5.54
DIET VISITS	81	78	79	233	0	ERR	0	1.36	3.39
HHA VISITS	9045	10358	9736	29139	28163	103%	118.47	116.32	4.84
TOTAL VISITS	34740	37616	35742	108098	107513	101%	475.33	420.96	4.96

STATE TOTALS — 2ND QTR

	OCT 88	NOV 88	DEC 88	TOTALS 2ND QTR	TARGET 2ND QTR	% TARGET MET	MID-YEAR TOTALS	% TARGET MET	MID-YEAR TARGET	MBO PROJECTED F.T.E.	F.T.E. 2ND QTR	2ND QTR AVG VISITS PER DAY
RN VISITS	15433	19702	17248	52383	58065	90%	109075	94%	116130	267.73	235.81	4.47
LPN VISITS	472	547	521	1540	2380	65%	3408	72%	4760	8.80	6.70	4.91
ALL NURSE VISITS	15905	20249	17769	53923	60445	89%	112483	93%	120890	276.53	242.51	4.48
HSW VISITS	814	1257	986	3057	3922	78%	6376	81%	7844	19.52	16.90	3.64
PT VISITS	3522	4932	4304	12758	10726	119%	25607	129%	19904	42.44	35.35	7.00
ST VISITS	340	620	553	1513	2173	70%	3361	77%	4346	9.20	5.20	6.24
OT VISITS	393	536	429	1358	2084	65%	3503	86%	4064	9.17	6.31	5.36
DIET VISITS	66	77	82	225	0	ERR	463	ERR	0	0	1.28	3.48
HHA VISITS	8418	9751	8922	27091	28163	96%	56230	100%	56326	118.47	118.12	4.60
TOTAL VISITS	29458	37422	33045	99925	107513	93%	208023	97%	215026	475.33	425.69	4.72

Spaulding Rehabilitation Hospital

125 Nashua Street
Boston, MA 02114

Beth Shea, OTR
Director of Occupational Therapy
(617) 720-6624

Type of setting:
Rehabilitation Hospital (Inpatient and Outpatient)

Number of beds:
284

Total number of FTEs for this setting:
78.5

Productivity standard (in hours per day):
OTR Entry Level: 5.5 hrs.
OTR Inter. Level: 5.5 hrs.
OTR Adv. Level: 4.0 hrs.
COTA Entry Level: 5.5 hrs.
COTA Inter. Level: 5.5 hrs.
COTA Adv. Level: 5.5 hrs.
Manager/Director: 0 hrs.
Fieldwork Supervisor/Coordinator: 0 hrs.

Spaulding uses 15-minute units for billing purposes, collecting data for their productivity reports from **Forms A** and **B**. Note that documentation is billable at 2 units per patient, per week. Also, home/school/clinic visits (including travel time) for a patient are billable, but they generally bill only for one of these types of visits, even if they do more.

The Weekly Productivity Report (**Form C**) is completed by each staff person. **Form D** and **Attachment A** are samples of weekly and yearly statistical reports respectively. Note that on Form D, if outpatient visits are down and weather is the reason, one can code that information.

Aides are currently assisting the OTRs and COTAs in group and maintenance activities. However, their use is under review and may change.

All forms and attachments in this section are courtesy of Spaulding Rehabilitation Hospital, Boston, MA. Reprinted with permission.

Form A

ADDRESSOGRAPH

SPAULDING REHABILITATION HOSPITAL

OCCUPATIONAL THERAPY

☐ INPATIENT

PLEASE INDICATE NUMBER OF UNITS FOR EACH ITEM.
ONE UNIT = 15 MINUTES.

THERAPIST / ASSISTANT: _____

		DATE	DATE	DATE	DATE
Evaluation	31610272				
Upper Extremity Evaluation	31610025				
Upper Extremity Positioning	31610041				
Upper Extremity Exercise	31610033				
Upper Extremity Functional Training	31610058				
Upper Extremity Physical Modalities	31610066				
Upper Extremity Neuromuscular Training	31610074				
Splinting	31610082				
Therapeutic Adaptations	31610090				
Activities of Daily Living Evaluation and Training	31610116				
Feeding / Swallowing Evaluation and Training	31610124				
Functional Mobility Evaluation and Training	31610132				
Homemaking Evaluation and Training	31610215				
Prevocational / Vocational Evaluation and Training	31610249				
Cognitive / Perceptual Evaluation and Training	31610348				
Computer-Assisted Therapy	31610355				
Trendscriber Evaluation	31610322				
Relaxation and Stress Management Training	31610223				
Supportive Treatment	31610314				
Home Evaluation	31610157				
Patient / Family Teaching	31610165				
Discharge Process	31610280				
Interagency Consult	31610298				
Treatment Documentation	31610306				
Group Programs	31610363				

SRH-324 REV. 10/89

BUSINESS OFFICE COPY

Managing Productivity in Occupational Therapy

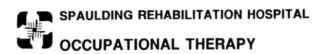

SPAULDING REHABILITATION HOSPITAL
OCCUPATIONAL THERAPY

OUTPATIENT

THERAPIST/
ASSISTANT: _____ Date _____

PLEASE CHECK BOX FOR UNIT(S) PROVIDED		DATE	DATE	DATE	DATE
1 Unit	31650013				
2 Units	31650021				
3 Units	31650039				
4 Units	31650047				
5 Units	31650054				
6 Units	31650062				
7 Units	31650070				
8 Units	31650088				
9 Units	31650096				
10 Units	31650104				
11 Units	31650112				
12 Units	31650120				

IF MORE THAN 12 INDIVIDUAL UNITS,

INDICATE TOTAL UNITS PROVIDED: _____ x $28.00 = _____   charge 31611122

MODALITIES	DATE	DATE	DATE	DATE
Evaluation				
Upper Extremity Treatment				
Therapeutic Adapt./Splinting				
ADL Eval./Training				
Feed/Swallow Eval./Training				
Func. Mobility Eval./Training				
Homemaking Eval./Training				
Prevoc./Voc. Eval./Training				
Cognitive/Percep. Eval./Training				
Home Evaluation				
Patient/Family Teaching				
Discharge Process				
Interagency Consult				
Group Program				

PLEASE INDICATE NUMBER OF UNITS FOR EACH ITEM. ONE UNIT = 15 MINUTES

GROUP UNITS PROVIDED: _____ x $23.00 = _____   charge 31611148

OCCUPATIONAL THERAPY DEPARTMENT

WEEKLY PRODUCTIVITY REPORT

Week starting Sunday _____   Ending Saturday _____

Name_____   ___OTR ___COTA ___OTA ___OTS

CHARGEABLE UNITS

	Mon	Tues	Wed	Thu	Fri
Total 1:1 Units					
Total units spent leading groups					
Daily total					

Weekly total_____units

NONCHARGEABLE UNITS

	Mon	Tue	Wed	Thu	Fri
Notes/Paperwork					
PCC					
Supervision/Staff					
Supervision/Student					
Inservice/OT					
Inservice/Other					
Staff Meeting					
Treatment Preparation					
Professional Conference					
Community Activity/Liaison					
Research					
Other(specify)					
TOTAL					

Weekly total _____units

Productivity Expectation
Chargeable Units - 100
Non chargeable Units - 50
Reasons for variance from norms:

_____ Earned Time for _____ Units

_____ Comp Time for _____ Units

_____ Patient Unavailable for _____ Units

_____ Other (please specify) _____ for _____ Units

For Supervisor Use
Discussed in supervision on _____ _____.
                              (Date)   (Supervisor)

Plan:_____ _____

Route as Follows: Staff therapist to Supervisor by Monday noon.
                  Supervisor to weekend Secretary by 4:30 Friday
                  Weekend Secretary to Assistant Director Monday
                  Assistant Director to Director (if significant)
                  Employee folder

SPAULDING REHABILITATION HOSPITAL
OCCUPATIONAL THERAPY DEPARTMENT WEEKLY STATISTICAL REPORT

Week Ending	# INPT Staff	Total Indivd. Units	Total Group Units	Total Wkend Units	Total Holiday Units	Total Aide Units	Avg. Units per Treating Therapist	# Outpt. Treating Staff	Total Individ. Units	Total Visits	Total Pts Seen	Total OPD Aide Units	Avg. Units per Treating Therapists

Comments:

SPAULDING REHABILITATION HOSPITAL
OCCUPATIONAL THERAPY DEPARTMENT

ANNUAL REPORT FISCAL YEAR 1989 - 1990

During FY 1988 - 1989, the Occupational Therapy Department evaluated and treated 3,398 in-patients and 268 out-patients for a total of 3,666 patients. The diagnostic breakdown is:

Diagnosis	Total	In-patients	Out-patients
STROKE	456	371	85
ORTHO.	404	390	14
MED./SURG.	205	204	1
ONC	230	225	5
CARD.	491	491	0
GEN. NEURO	102	72	30
HEAD INJURY	212	146	66
ETOH	286	286	0
PUL.	270	268	2
AMP.	79	79	0
PAIN	308	302	6
ARTHRITIS	75	62	13
MAJOR FRACTURE	373	372	1
MUSCLE DISEASE	30	26	4
SCI	46	39	7
SAB	48	47	1
PEDIATRICS	48	18	30
OTHER	3	0	3
TOTAL	3666	3398	268

15 MINUTE TREATMENT UNITS

MONTH	IN-PT.	OUT-PT.	WK. END	TOTAL
OCTOBER	18,391	1,823	1,236	21,450
NOVEMBER	20,455	1,831	994	23,280
DECEMBER	19,847	1,501	1,157	22,505
JANUARY	21,604	1,622	835	24,061
FEBRUARY	20,065	1,497	1,187	22,749
MARCH	23,127	1,517	1,495	26,139
APRIL	21,027	1,471	1,192	23,690
MAY	22,834	1,765	1,037	25,636
JUNE	21,003	1,676	1,045	23,724
JULY	24,356	1,574	1,146	27,076
AUGUST	25,157	1,897	973	28,027
SEPTEMBER	21,262	1,555	1,404	24,221
TOTAL	259,128	19,729	13,701	292,558

CLINICS	NUMBER OF PATIENTS
POST POLIO	28
PEDIATRIC	81
DRIVING EVALS	123

Rehabilitation Hospital of the Pacific

226 North Kuakini Street
Honolulu, HI 96817

Virginia Tully, OTR
Director of Therapies and Ancillary Services
(808) 531-3511

Type of setting:
Rehabilitation Hospital—Inpatient

Number of beds:
70

Total number of FTEs for this setting:
21

Productivity standard (in hours per day):
OTR Entry Level: 6.75 hrs.
OTR Inter. Level: N/A
OTR Adv. Level: 4.0 hrs.
COTA Entry Level: 8.0 hrs.
COTA Inter. Level: N/A
COTA Adv. Level: N/A
Manager/Director: 0 hrs.
Fieldwork Supervisor/Coordinator: N/A

Type of setting:
Outpatient, Hand, and Work Hardening

Number of beds:
N/A

Total number of FTEs for this setting:
14
3.5 Outpatient
6.5 Hand
4.0 Work Hardening

Productivity standard (in hours per day):
OTR Entry Level: 6.0 hrs.
OTR Inter. Level: N/A
OTR Adv. Level: 4.0 hrs.

This rehabilitation hospital has established a productivity standard for hand, work-hardening, and outpatient services that is slightly less than the inpatient services. The hospital bills by 15-minute units of time.

The Inpatient Charge Slip (**Form A**) schedule is generated by the Patient Schedule Sheet (not shown). The therapist can make changes on the right hand side to the schedule, including staff changes and reasons for "late" or "no show." "No show" is defined as absence from therapy. "Late" is a decrease in therapy session or being late for the therapy session. The total hours for each code of no show/late are calculated on a daily, weekly, and monthly basis and appear in the Inpatient Treatment Statistics. The inpatient treatment statistics report provides information on each clinic by weekday, weekend, and holidays. (A weekly summary of the kind of data collected is shown on **Attachment A**.) The information on this report is generated by the charges and provides patient, not staff, data. The therapists' data are reported on **Attachment B** by department and on **Attachment C** by individual therapists.

All forms and attachments in this section are courtesy of the Rehabilitation Hospital of the Pacific, Honolulu, HI. Reprinted with permission.

Continues on next page

COTA Entry Level: 9.0 hrs (work hardening only)
COTA Inter. Level: N/A
COTA Adv. Level: N/A
Manager/Director: N/A
Fieldwork Supervisor/Coordinator: N/A

REHABILITATION HOSPITAL OF THE PACIFIC   RMBED 201-1

PATIENT NAME		PATIENT NO. 0188896A	IN	OUT	DATE 3/06/91	DEPT./FLOOR 638	PAGE 1 OF 63	ADD
			X					

#	✓	TIME (FROM)	—	TIME (TO)	THERAPIST	ASS'T.
1		9 : 00	—	10 : 00	685	
2		3 : 00	—	3 : 30	685	
3		:	—	:		
4		:	—	:		
5		:	—	:		
6		:	—	:		

OVERRIDE

#	NS CODE	TIME (FROM)	—	TIME (TO)	THERAPIST	ASS'T.
1		7 : 30	—	8 : 00	723	
2		9 : 30	—	10 : 00	685	
3	F	3 : 00	—	3 : 45	685	
4		:	—	:		
5		:	—	:		
6		:	—	:		

PRI INS - MEDICARE

DESCRIPTION	UNITS	DP	CODE	DESCRIPTION	UNITS	DP	CODE	DESCRIPTION	UNITS	DP	CODE	DESCRIPTION	UNITS	DP	CODE
EVALUATIONS				EA. ADD'L 15 MINS.		12	72604-02	**HOME ASSESSMENT**				**SUPPLIES**			
1ST 15 MINS.		1	72400-5	**GROUP THERAPY**				10 MI. RADIUS, 1ST 15 MINS.		24	72880-8				
EA. ADD'L 15 MINS.		2	72401-3	1ST 15 MINS.		13	97430-3	EA. ADD'L 15 MINS.		25	72885-7				
DRIVING				EA. ADD'L 15 MINS.		14	97431-1	10 MI. + RADIUS, 1ST 15 MINS.		26	72890-7				
1ST 15 MINS.		3	72609-1	**DRIVER TRAINING**				EA. ADD'L 15 MINS.		27	72895-6				
EA. ADD'L 15 MINS.		4	72610-9	SIM. TMG., 1ST 15 MINS.		15	72611-7	**PATIENT / HOME INTEGRATION**							
THERAPY				EA. ADD'L 15 MINS.		16	72612-5	10 MI. RADIUS, 1ST 15 MINS.		30	72900-4				
ADL. 1ST 15 MINS.	2	5	72600-0	ON-THE-ROAD BTW TMG.				EA. ADD'L 15 MINS.		31	72901-2				
EA. ADD'L 15 MINS.	2	6	72602-6	1ST 15 MINS.		18	72613-3	10 MI. + RADIUS, 1ST 15 MINS.		32	72902-0				
CLINIC, FIRST SESSION				EA. ADD'L 15 MINS.		19	72614-1	EA. ADD'L 15 MINS.		33	72903-8				
1ST 15 MINS.		7	72603-4	**FAMILY CONFERENCE**				**ORTHOTICS TRAINING**							
EA. ADD'L 15 MINS.		8	72604-2	1ST 15 MINS.		20	72775-0	1ST 15 MINS.		34	97500-3				
SECOND SESSION				EA. ADD'L 15 MINS.		21	72780-0	EA. ADD'L 15 MINS.		35	97501-1				
1ST 15 MINS.		9	72603-4	**FAMILY ORIENTATION**				**ORTHO / PROSTH. FABRICATION**							
EA. ADD'L 15 MINS.		10	72604-2	1ST 15 MINS.	1	22	72800-6	INITIAL 15 MIN.		76	97512-8				
THIRD SESSION 1ST 15 MINS.		11	72603-4	EA. ADD'L 15 MINS.	2	23	72801-4	EA. ADD'L 15 MINS.		77	97513-6				

WORKER'S COMPENSATION

DESCRIPTION	UNITS	DP	CODE	DESCRIPTION	UNITS	DP	CODE	DESCRIPTION	UNITS	DP	CODE	DESCRIPTION	UNITS	DP	CODE
EVALUATION				**COMBO PROCED / MODAL**				**BTE WORK SIMULATOR**				**SUPPLIES**			
INITIAL 15 MIN.		38	97400-6	INITIAL 15 MIN.		48	97418-8	INITIAL 15 MIN.		78	97440-2				
EACH ADD'L. 15 MIN.		74	97401-4	EACH ADD'L. 15 MIN.		49	97419-6	EACH ADD'L. 15 MIN.		79	97441-0				
RE-EVALUATION				**GROUP SESSION / OTR SUPERVISE**				**HOME ASSESSMENT**							
INITIAL 15 MIN.		75	97402-2	INITIAL 15 MIN.		50	97423-8	10 MI. RADIUS, 1ST 15 MINS.		24	72880-8				
EACH ADD'L. 15 MIN.		41	97403-0	EACH ADD'L. 15 MIN.		51	97424-6	EACH ADD'L. 15 MIN.		25	72885-7				
THERAPEUTIC EXERCISE				**ORTHO / PROSTH. TRAINING**				10 MI. + RADIUS, 1ST 15 MINS.		26	72890-7				
INITIAL 15 MIN.		42	97405-5	INITIAL 15 MIN.		52	97510-2	EACH ADD'L. 15 MIN.		27	72895-6				
EACH ADD'L. 15 MIN.		43	97406-3	EACH ADD'L. 15 MIN.		53	97511-0	**PATIENT / HOME INTEGRATION**							
MODALITIES				**ORTHO / PROSTH. FABRICATION**				10 MI. RADIUS, 1ST 15 MINS.		30	72900-4				
ONE MODALITY		44	97414-7	INITIAL 15 MIN.		76	97512-8	EACH ADD'L. 15 MIN.		31	72901-2				
TWO MODALITIES		45	97415-4	EACH ADD'L. 15 MIN.		77	97513-6	10 MI. + RADIUS, 1ST 15 MINS.		32	72902-0				
ONE PROCEDURE				**ACT OF DAILY LIVING**				EACH ADD'L. 15 MIN.		33	72903-8				
INITIAL 15 MIN.		46	97416-2	INITIAL 15 MIN.		58	97410-5								
EACH ADD'L. 15 MIN.		47	97417-0	EACH ADD'L. 15 MIN.		59	97411-3								

NO-SHOW CODES ▶

I - ILLNESS	C - CONFERENCE / THERAPIST	O - OTHER APPT.	T - TOILET
F - FATIGUE	L - LATE FROM PREVIOUS THERAPY	R - REFUSAL	PR - PERSONAL BUSINESS
SF - STAFF	NA - NOT APPLICABLE	DC - DISCHARGE	M - MEDICAL

INPATIENT TREATMENT STATISTICS
For 3/09/91 (Weekly)

FOR - OT
(APD) - AVERAGE PER DAY

	MONDAY THRU FRIDAY			WEEKENDS & HOLIDAYS		
OCCUPATIONAL THERAPY	A-2	A-3	A-4	A-2	A-3	A-4
CENSUS:						
PATIENT COUNT (APU)						
TREATMENT COUNT;						
NUMBER TREATED (APD)						
TREATMENT SESSIONS:						
UNSCHEDULED						
SCHEDULED						
UNSCH/SCHED TOTAL						
UNSCH/SCH (APD)						
ACTUAL						
ACTUAL (APD)						
ACTUAL AVG HRS BY SESSIONS:						
FOR REPORTING PERIOD						
REVENUE:						
THERAPY						
SUPPLY						
OTHER						
NO SHOWS:						
CONFERENCE/THERAPIST						
DISCHARGE						
FATIGUE						
ILLNESS						
LATE FR.PREV.THERAPY						
MEDICAL						
OTHER APPOINTMENT						
PERSONAL BUSINESS						
REFUSAL						
STAFF						
TOILET						
(NOT APPLICABLE)						
TOTAL						

NOTE: A-2, A-3, A-4 = Clinic Sites

DATE 2/07/91
FOR DIR. THERAPY/ANC SERV., PROGRAMS

SUMMARY OF INPATIENT PRODUCTIVITY STATS
FISCAL YR-91   MONTH-JANUARY

ID-M121HH

OCCUPATIONAL THERAPY

STANDARD IS   BILL HRS/STAFF-6.70   TOTAL STAFF HRS-3286.86

	OCT	NOV	DEC	JAN	FEB	MAR	APR	MAY	JUNE	JULY	AUG	SEPT	AVG
BILLED HOURS	2617.50	2458.75	1905.75	2179.50	.00	.00	.00	.00	.00	.00	.00	.00	2290.38
STAFF HOURS	3539.50	3353.00	2968.75	3420.00	.00	.00	.00	.00	.00	.00	.00	.00	3320.31
BILL HRS/STAFF	5.92	5.87	5.14	5.10	.00	.00	.00	.00	.00	.00	.00	.00	5.52
EVALUATION – A2	42	41	28	37	0	0	0	0	0	0	0	0	37.0
A3	29	35	31	29	0	0	0	0	0	0	0	0	31.0
A4	37	34	27	38	0	0	0	0	0	0	0	0	34.0

FOR - OT
ID-MISO5H

3/06/91   7.58.44   PAGE   4

THERAPIST HOURS
BY- DEPARTMENT/THERAPISTS

FROM 2/17/91 TO 3/02/91

DEPARTMENT- 638   OCCUP THERAPY

THERAPISTS

EMP#	NON-WKD HOURS	HOURS WORKED	OTHER	DAP	MLT	SCP	STK	ARP	HIP	PCI
000	.00	6.50	.00	4.00	.00	.00	2.50	.00	.00	.00
761	.00	24.00	5.25	3.50	.00	.00	11.50	.00	3.75	.00
257	.00	.00	2.75-	.00	.00	.00	2.75	.00	.00	.00
414	8.00	72.00	20.99	1.25	.50	15.38	33.88	.00	.00	.00
818 *	.00	8.25	4.75	.00	.00	.00	3.50	.00	.00	.00
566	.00	15.00	2.25	2.17	.00	1.50	7.08	.00	2.00	.00
616	8.00	72.00	25.24	.88	.00	.00	45.88	.00	.00	.00
302	12.00	67.25	47.75	6.50	.00	.00	4.75	.00	8.25	.00
823	16.00	64.00	26.75	35.25	.00	.00	.00	.00	2.00	.00
503	24.00	56.00	29.00	.50	.00	3.75	22.75	.00	.00	.00
626 *	.00	14.75	11.75	1.00	.00	.00	2.00	.00	.00	.00
387	.00	.00	.51-	.00	.00	.13	.38	.00	.00	.00
444	8.00	65.50	31.75	12.25	.00	.00	2.00	.00	19.50	.00
638	12.00	43.00	19.75	26.75	.00	.00	.00	.00	1.50	.00
723	8.00	72.00	25.75	.00	.00	.00	46.25	.00	.00	.00
290	.00	8.00	1.25	.00	.00	.00	4.00	.00	2.75	.00
676	16.00	64.00	31.00	4.50	.00	5.58	22.92	.00	.00	.00
662	8.00	72.00	32.00	6.21	.00	.00	33.79	.00	.00	.00
788	.00	8.00	1.25	1.00	.00	.00	5.25	.00	.50	.00
739	.00	8.00	1.25	1.00	.00	2.00	3.75	.00	.00	.00
523	18.00	62.00	43.25	.00	.00	.00	18.75	.00	.00	.00
686	6.50	52.25	21.00	12.31	.00	1.00	16.94	.00	1.00	.00
685	8.00	72.00	22.25	.00	.00	.00	49.75	.00	.00	.00
412	16.00	64.00	41.75	2.00	.50	12.75	7.00	.00	1.00	.00
780	8.00	71.75	27.75	2.25	.00	1.00	40.75	.00	.00	.00
629 *	.00	7.00	5.30	.50	.00	1.00	.50	.00	.00	.00
590	8.00	62.00	26.49	11.88	.00	.00	22.63	.00	1.00	.00
025	16.00	64.00	25.25	.00	.00	16.50	22.25	.00	.00	.00
610	16.00	56.00	18.75	12.75	.00	.00	24.50	.00	.00	.00
502	8.00	72.00	30.75	33.50	.00	.00	7.75	.00	.00	.00
815 *	.00	14.50	9.00	.25	.00	.75	4.50	.00	.00	.00
692 *	2.00	6.00	1.00	1.00	.00	.00	4.00	.00	.00	.00
624	.00	7.50	1.25	1.75	.00	.00	4.50	.00	.00	.00
327	56.00	24.00	23.00	.00	.00	.00	1.00	.00	.00	.00
793	8.00	72.00	29.49	17.63	.00	.00	6.00	.00	18.88	.00
SUBTOTAL HOURS	290.50	1452.25	640.45	202.58	1.00	60.34	485.75	.00	62.13	.00
%			640.45	24.95%	.12%	7.43%	59.84%	.00%	7.65%	.00%

OTHER HOURS   16.00 ... 640.45   159.79   .77   47.59   383.25   .00   48.99   .00

NO INP.CHRGS FOR-

EMP#	NON-WKD	WORKED	OTHER	DAP	MLT	SCP	STK	ARP	HIP	PCI
498	16.00	64.00		15.97	.08	4.76	38.30	.00	4.90	.00
706	.00	.00		.00	.00	.00	.00	.00	.00	.00
202 *	.00	15.50		3.87	.02	1.15	9.28	.00	1.19	.00
396	.00	.00		.00	.00	.00	.00	.00	.00	.00
111	15.00	64.00		15.97	.08	4.76	38.30	.00	4.90	.00

Children's Memorial Hospital

2300 Children's Plaza
Chicago, IL 60614

Kathleen Zahner, OTR/L
Supervisor, Occupational Therapy
(312) 880-6920

Type of setting:
Acute Pediatric Hospital

Number of beds:
265

Total number of FTEs for this setting:
7

Productivity standard (in hours per day):
OTR Entry Level: 4.75 hrs.
OTR Inter. Level: 4.75 hrs.
OTR Adv. Level: 4.75 hrs.
COTA Entry Level: N/A
COTA Inter. Level: N/A
COTA Adv. Level: N/A
Manager/Director: 2 hrs.
Fieldwork Supervisor/Coordinator: 3 hrs.
Orthotic Supervisor-OT: 5 hrs.

Type of setting:
Outpatient

Number of beds:
N/A

Total number of FTEs for this setting:
5

Productivity standard (in hours per day):
OTR Entry Level: 7 hrs.
OTR Inter. Level: 7 hrs.
OTR Adv. Level: 7 hrs.

Inpatient care is generally billed in 10-minute units and outpatient care in 30- to 60-minute units. In the Orthotic Department the type of orthosis determines how billing is done. There can be a per-item charge, or it can be done by 10-minute units. Productivity data are gathered from **Form A** and the therapist attendance sheet. Note in OT column the descriptors *Consultation* and *2nd Opinion*. These are 10-minute units of which the former is billable and the latter is not, but is used to track productivity data.

Performance appraisals for staff are based partly on predetermined productivity standards. These standards are in percentages and are obtained from the following formula:

$$\text{Volume} \div 6 \div \text{hours worked} = \%$$

Form A is courtesy of Children's Memorial Hospital, Chicago, IL. Reprinted with permission.

Continues on next page

COTA Entry Level: N/A
COTA Inter. Level: N/A
COTA Adv. Level: N/A
Manager/Director (Treating Supervisor): 7 hrs. (more or less, depending on the week)
Fieldwork Supervisor/Coordinator: N/A

the children's memorial hospital
2300 children's plaza • chicago, illinois 60614
OUTPATIENT REGISTRATION

PT	PATIENT ACCOUNT NO.	ALC	MED. REC. NO.		DATE SERVICE	REG. BY

PATIENT NAME (LAST, FIRST)		BIRTHDATE	AGE	SEX	RC	REL	ACC/INJ 0	VISIT TYPE

PATIENT LOCAL ADDRESS	CITY	STATE	ZIP	PATIENT LOCAL PHONE

PATIENT PERMANENT ADDRESS (IF DIFFERENT)	CITY	STATE	ZIP	PATIENT PERMANENT PHONE

FATHER'S NAME (LAST, FIRST, MIDDLE INITIAL)	MOTHER'S NAME (LAST, FIRST, MAIDEN)	STEP PARENT/LEGAL GUARDIAN (LAST, FIRST)

GUARANTOR NAME	GUARANTOR ADDRESS

CITY, STATE	ZIP	GUARANTOR PHONE	RELATIONSHIP	GUARANTOR SOC. SEC. NO.	GUARANTOR OCCUPATION

GUARANTOR EMPLOYER NAME	GUARANTOR EMPLOYER ADDRESS	CITY, STATE	ZIP	GUARANTOR EMPLOYER PHONE

F/C	THIRD PARTY NAME	SUBSCRIBER NAME	CO. NO.	PLAN NO.	GROUP NO.	POLICY NO.

REL. OF SUBSCRIBER	RECIPIENT NAME	RECIPIENT NO.	CLINIC NAME KIDS THERAPY-L. PARK	CLINIC NO. 83

ATT. PHY. NO.	ATTENDING PHYSICIAN NAME

REFER PHY. NO.	REFERRING PHYSICIAN/CLINIC	REFERRING PHONE	REFERRING PHYSICIAN/CLINIC ADDRESS

FAMILY PHY. NO.	FAMILY PHYSICIAN/CLINIC	FAMILY PHONE	FAMILY PHYSICIAN/CLINIC ADDRESS

PRIMARY DIAGNOSIS	HMO AUTH.	ADMIT	PHYSICIAN FEE

QTY.	CODE	TEST	$	¢	QTY.	CODE	TEST	$	¢	QTY.	CODE	TEST	$	¢
		355- P.T.					355- O.T.					MATERIAL		
	57XX	OP EVAL-30				57XX	OP EVAL-30				0300	ADAPTAFOAM MATERIAL		
	58XX	OP EVAL-60				58XX	OP EVAL-60							
	59XX	OP EVAL-90				59XX	OP EVAL-90				08XX	SPLINT MATERIAL		
	32XX	EQUIP EVAL				32XX	EQUIP EVAL				1400	WALKER		
	30XX	CNX PRE-OP EVAL				72XX	SPLINT FAB				1900	MISCELLANEOUS		
						39XX	BAYLEY>12MO							
						40XX	BAYLEY<12MO							
	63XX	OP TX-30				43XX	V.M.I.							
	64XX	OP TX-60												
	67XX	OP TX-90				44XX	M.F.V.P.							
						47XX	T.V.P.S.							
	0362	ADAPTAFOAM FIT				48XX	T.V.M.S.							
	52XX	SPLINT MOD				49XX	S.C.S.I.T.							
	56XX	CASTING												
	73XX	EQUIP TRNG				50XX	BRUININKS							
	74XX	EQUIP FAB				51XX	BRUININKS-SHRT							
	68XX	CNS ORTHO REHAB				69XX	M.A.P.							
	86XX	AGENCY VISIT<3												
	87XX	AGENCY VISIT>3				78XX	HAWAII							
	98XX	2ND OPINION/SU				79XX	PEABODY							
						80XX	PEABODY F/G ONLY							
	01XX	BEDSIDE												
	99XX	CONSULTATION				81XX	DIGANGI-BURKE							
		SUPPLIES				63XX	OPTX-30							
						64XX	OPTX-60							
	0300	ADAPTAFOAM MAT				67XX	OPTX-90							
	08XX	SPLINT MATL												
	1400	WALKER				0362	ADAPTAFOAM FIT							
	19XX	MISCELLANEOUS				52XX	SPLINT MOD							
						56XX	CASTING							
						73XX	EQUIP TRNG			*****	FOLLOW-UP CHARGES MAY APPEAR ON FINAL BILLING			
						74XX	EQUIP FAB							
						68XX	CNS ORTHO REHB							
						8600	AGENCY VST<3HR							
						8700	AGENCY VST>3HR				VISIT CODE			
						98XX	2ND OPINION SUP				TOTAL			
						01XX	BEDSIDE				DIFFERENTIAL			
						99XX	CONSULTATION				AMOUNT PAID			
											BALANCE DUE			

Section 3:
Productivity Data

Ira T. Silvergleit, MA, MS
Director
Research Information & Evaluation Department
American Occupational Therapy Association

1990 AOTA Member Data Survey

The following tables were generated from responses to the 1990 AOTA Member Data Survey. The two questions that elicited the data were:

- How many hours a day do you spend in direct patient/client service?
- What is the average number of patients/clients seen per day?

The data were analyzed separately for OTRs and COTAs, as well as by primary work function (administration, supervision, direct service personnel, etc.), primary work setting (general hospital, nursing home, etc.), and primary patient age range. The term *primary* denotes that respondents could give more than one answer per question; only the first answer given is used for these analyses. It does not imply that this is the only work setting or the only health problem seen or the only age range treated.

These results are for informational purposes only. **They are not intended and should not be regarded as standards of productivity.** The AOTA disclaims any intention to dictate norms of productivity to the profession; these results are simply what was found among those occupational therapists and occupational therapy assistants who chose to reply to these items on the membership survey. The data are released as a service to the field. Many factors, such as types of caseloads, staffing levels, documentation requirements, types of assessments, etc., all influence what productivity might be expected in a given facility or department or from an individual therapist.

The statistics reported are the *mean* (the arithmetic average) and *mode* (the response given most frequently). In order to give readers an indication of the *range* of responses, selected *percentiles* are shown. Percentiles are the values below which given percentages of cases fall. For example, the 25th percentile value is the value that, if all the responses were listed from smallest to largest, would fall a quarter of the way along the list. The 50th percentile is the value that divides the distribution of responses in half; half the values would fall below and half above. The 50th percentile is also known as the *median*.

Breakdowns with insufficient numbers of respondents are excluded from the tables. Therefore, not every category is included in each table.

List of Tables in Section 3

Table 3.1 Number of patients/clients treated daily by full-time personnel in direct patient service.

Patients	OTRs	COTAs
Mean	9.3	10.8
Median	8	9
Mode	8	10

Source: 1990 AOTA Member Data Survey

Table 3.2 Daily hours in direct patient/client service for full-time personnel in direct patient service.

Hours	OTRs	COTAs
Mean	5.8	5.9
Median	6	6
Mode	6	6

Source: 1990 AOTA Member Data Survey

Table 3.3 Number of patients treated daily by primary work setting for OTRs employed full-time in direct service.

Setting	Mean	Mode	Percentiles						
			10	25	33.3	50	66.6	75	90
Community Mental Health Center	14.6	20	5	8	10	13	20	20	27
Day Care Program	10.8	8	5	6	7	8	12	14	20
HMO/PPO/IPA	10.3	9	6	8	9	10	11	12	15
Home Health Agency	6	5	4	5	5	5	6	7	9
General Hospital—NICU	7.7	6	5	6	6	7	8	9	11
General Hospital—Psych	15.0	15	8	10	12	15	17	20	25
General Hospital—Rehab	7.3	5	4	5	5	6	8	9	12
General Hospital—Other	8.9	8	5	6	7	8	10	10	14
Pediatric Hospital	7	6	5	6	6	7	7	8	10
Psychiatric Hospital	15.9	20	6	10	12	15	20	20	25
Outpatient Clinic	9.1	8	5	6	7	8	10	12	15
Rehabilitation Center/Hospital	7.9	6	5	6	6	7	8	9	12
School System	9.6	10	6	7	8	9	10	11	15
Skilled Nursing Facility/ICF	8.6	6	5	6	7	8	9	10	13
Sheltered Workshop	10.2	7	5	6	7	8	9	12	24
Vocational/Prevocational Program	7.6	3	2	3	4	6	10	12	15

Source: 1990 AOTA Member Data Survey

Managing Productivity in Occupational Therapy

Table 3.4 Number of patients treated daily by primary work setting for COTAs employed full-time in direct service.

| Setting | Mean | Mode | Percentiles | | | | | | |
			10	25	33.3	50	66.6	75	90
Community Mental Health Center	15.7	4	4	10	11	15	20	22	30
Day Care Program	15.2	20	4	9	13	16	20	20	26
Home Health Agency	5.5	6	2	4	5	6	6	6	9
General Hospital—Psych	17.2	10	8	10	12	16	20	22	29
General Hospital—Rehab	8.1	5	4	5	6	8	10	10	12
General Hospital—Other	10.3	8	5	6	7	8	11	13	16
Pediatric Hospital	7.9	6	—	5	6	7	9	10	—
Psychiatric Hospital	17.1	20	8	12	14	17	20	22	27
Outpatient Clinic	10.4	12	5	6	7	9	12	12	20
Rehabilitation Center/Hospital	9.2	6	5	6	7	8	10	10	15
School System	9.4	10	6	7	8	9	10	11	14
Skilled Nursing Facility/ICF	10.5	6	5	6	7	9	11	12	20
Sheltered Workshop	11.5	10	6	7	8	10	10	13	27
Vocational/Prevocational Program	13.0	10	4	6	7	10	12	20	30

Source: 1990 AOTA Member Data Survey

Table 3.5 Number of patients treated daily by primary work setting for OTRs employed full-time as administrators.

Setting	Mean	Mode	Percentiles						
			10	25	33.3	50	66.6	75	90
Community Mental Health Center	7.5	1	1	1	2	3	13.3	15	20
Home Health Agency	4.3	1	1	2	2	3	4	4.8	11.8
General Hospital—Psych	10	15	3	5	6	10	13	15	18.4
General Hospital—Rehab	4.6	4	2	2.8	3	4	5	6.3	8
General Hospital—Other	5.9	4	1	3	3	5	7	8	12
Pediatric Hospital	3.3	2	1	2	2	3	4	4.3	7
Psychiatric Hospital	9.2	10	1	3	4	8	10	12	20
Outpatient Clinic	6.2	1	1	2	3	5	8.3	10	13
Rehabilitation Center/Hospital	5.7	2	1	2	2	4	6	8	12
School System	7.3	5	1.7	4	4.3	5.5	8	10	12.3
Skilled Nursing Facility/ICF	6.1	2	2	3	3.3	5	7	8	12
Sheltered Workshop	4.4	2	—	2	2	4	6	6	—

Source: 1990 AOTA Member Data Survey

Managing Productivity in Occupational Therapy

Table 3.6 Number of patients treated daily by primary work setting for OTRs employed full-time as supervisors.

Setting	Mean	Mode	Percentiles						
			10	25	33.3	50	66.6	75	90
Home Health Agency	3.8	2	1.1	2	2	3.5	4.3	5	9.5
General Hospital—Psych	9.8	3	3	3	4.7	8.5	12	15	22.3
General Hospital—Rehab	5.4	3	2	3	3	4	5.6	6	9.8
General Hospital—Other	6.1	4	2	3.3	4	5	6	8	12
Pediatric Hospital	4.7	3	2.3	3	3.3	4.5	5.7	6	7.7
Psychiatric Hospital	9.6	8	2	4	5	8	10	15	17.4
Outpatient Clinic	5.3	4	—	3	4	5	5.7	7.5	—
Rehabilitation Center/Hospital	4.9	2	2	2	3	4	5	6.3	9
School System	5.6	3	2	3	3	4.5	6	7.8	10
Skilled Nursing Facility/ICF	6.6	5	3	4	5	5.5	7	8	11.8

Source: 1990 AOTA Member Data Survey

Table 3.7 Number of patients treated daily by primary work setting for OTRs employed full-time as consultants.

Setting	Mean	Mode	Percentiles						
			10	25	33.3	50	66.6	75	90
General Hospital—Psych	9.8	2	—	2.5	4	7	15	15.8	—
General Hospital—Other	10.4	10	5	6	7	9	11.3	13	20
Rehabilitation Center/Hospital	7.1	2	2	3	4	6	9	12	13.4
School System	8	10	4	5	6	7	9.9	10	12
Skilled Nursing Facility/ICF	7.4	4	3	4	5	7	8	9.5	14.4

Source: 1990 AOTA Member Data Survey

Table 3.8 Number of patients treated daily by primary health problems for OTRs employed full-time in direct patient service.

Health Problem	Mean	Mode	Percentiles						
			10	25	33.3	50	66.6	75	90
Alzheimer Disease	13	8	5.2	7.3	8	10	15	20	21.9
Arthritis/Collagen Disorders	7.6	5	4	5	6	7	8	9	12
Back Injury	8.6	6	4	5	6	7	10	10	15
Burn	8	10	3.6	6	7	8	10	10	12
Cancer	7.5	5	4.4	5	5	7	7.3	8	14.8
Cardiopulmonary Diseases	7.9	6	4.1	5	6	7.5	10	10	12
Cerebral Palsy	8.5	8	5	6	7	8	9	10	12
Congenital Anomalies	6.9	5	4	5	5.7	7	8	9	10
CVA Hemiplegia	7.7	6	5	6	6	7	8	9	12
Developmental Delay	8.7	8	5	6	7	8	10	10	14
Feeding Disorders	6.6	4	4	5	5.7	6.5	7.3	8	10
Fracture	8.2	6	5	6	6	8	9	10	12
Hand Injury	10.8	10	6	8	8	10	12	13	16
Learning Disability	9.6	10	6	7	8	9	10	11	14.8
Neuro/Muscular Disorder	7.7	6	3.5	5.3	6	6.5	8	9.8	14.5
Respiratory Disease	8.2	7	4.4	7	7	8	9.3	10	11.6
Spinal Cord Injury	6.2	5	4	5	5	6	7	7	8.7
Traumatic Brain Injury	7.2	6	4	5	6	7	8	8	11
Visual Disability	9.7	10	4	5.8	6	8.5	10	11.3	21.3
Adjustment Disorders	15	12	6	8	11.3	15	18.6	20	25.3
Affective Disorders	15.6	15	8	10	12	15	17.8	20	25
Alcohol/Substance Use Disorders	17.6	15	8	12	13.3	15	20	25	30
Eating Disorders	13	20	6	7	8	13	20	20	20
Mental Retardation	9.5	8	4	7	7.9	9	10	11	15
Organic Mental Disorders	13.5	15	5.5	8	9	12	15	16	25
Personality Disorders	14.5	10	6.8	9.3	10	12	15	19.5	27.3
Schizophrenic Disorders	15.8	20	8	10	12	15	20	20	25
Other Mental Health Disorders	11.9	10	5	8	9.3	10	14.3	15	20.2
Other	7.8	6	4	5.5	6	7	8.6	9.5	13.4

Source: 1990 AOTA Member Data Survey

Managing Productivity in Occupational Therapy

Table 3.9 Number of patients treated daily by primary health problems for COTAs employed full-time in direct patient service.

Health Problem	Mean	Mode	Percentiles						
			10	25	33.3	50	66.6	75	90
Alzheimer Disease	13.8	20	4	6	8.7	12	20	20	25
Back Injury	9.8	10	4.1	6	6	9.5	11.3	12	17.8
Cerebral Palsy	8.6	8	4.4	6	7	8	9.3	10	12
CVA Hemiplegia	8.9	6	5	6	6	8	10	10	14
Developmental Delay	9.1	8	5	6.5	7.6	8	10	11	13
Hand Injury	11.8	8	7	8	9	10	12	13	20.6
Learning Disability	10	10	5	8	9	10	10	12	15
Neuro/Muscular Disorder	11.6	8	—	8	8	9	10.7	12	—
Spinal Cord Injury	6.9	8	2	4	4.7	6.5	8	8	14.3
Traumatic Brain Injury	8.7	6	4	6	6	8	10	11	13.8
Adjustment Disorders	14.1	10	7.6	10	10	12	16	19	21.4
Affective Disorders	18.8	15	9.8	13.5	15	19	20.9	24	30
Alcohol/Substance Use Disorders	15.4	10	6	10	10	15	18.6	20	28
Mental Retardation	12.1	10	6	8	9	10	12	14	22.1
Organic Mental Disorders	16.3	12	7.2	12	12	15	18	21.5	30
Personality Disorders	18.9	20	10.2	13.5	14.7	20	21	23.5	29.5
Schizophrenic Disorders	15.6	15	5	10	12	15	19.9	20	25
Other Mental Health Disorders	19.2	20	6.3	13.5	16.3	20	23	25.8	29.8

Source: 1990 AOTA Member Data Survey

Table 3.10 Number of patients treated daily by age range for OTRs employed full-time in direct patient service.

Age Range of Patients	Mean	Mode	Percentiles						
			10	25	33.3	50	66.6	75	90
Less than 3 years	7.1	6	4	5	6	7	8	8	11
3 to 5 years	9	8	5	7	7	8	10	10	14
6 to 12 years	9.5	10	6	7	8	9	10	11	15
13 to 18 years	11.5	10	5	7	8	10	12	14	20
19 to 64 years	10.5	8	5	6	7	9	12	13	20
65 to 74 years	7.8	6	5	6	6	7	8	9	12
75 to 84 years	7.8	6	5	6	6	7	8	9	12
84+ years	9.2	5	5	6	6	8	10	10.8	15

Source: 1990 AOTA Member Data Survey

Table 3.11 Number of patients treated daily by age range for COTAs employed full-time in direct patient service.

Age Range of Patients	Mean	Mode	Percentiles						
			10	25	33.3	50	66.6	75	90
Less than 3 years	8.4	4	4	5	6	8	9	10.5	15.8
3 to 5 years	8.9	10	5	7	8	8	10	10	12.2
6 to 12 years	9.7	10	6	7	8	10	10	11	14.5
13 to 18 years	11.3	8	6.4	8	8	10	12.3	15	19.2
19 to 64 years	12.4	10	5	7	8	10	13	16	25
65 to 74 years	9.2	6	5	6	6	8	10	10	15
75 to 84 years	10.1	8	5	6	7	8	10	12	19.1
84+ years	12	9	5	7.5	9	10	13	15	21.9

Source: 1990 AOTA Member Data Survey

Table 3.12 Hours per day in direct patient service by primary work setting for OTRs employed full-time in direct patient service.

Setting	Mean	Mode	Percentiles						
			10	25	33.3	50	66.6	75	90
Community Mental Health Center	4.7	5	3	4	4	5	5	5.5	6.5
Day Care Program	5.4	5	4	5	5	5.5	6	6	7
HMO IPA	6.4	6.5	4.7	5.7	6	6.5	7	7.3	8
Home Health Agency	5.6	5	4	4.5	5	5.5	6.3	6.5	8
General Hospital—NICU	5.7	6.5	4	5	5.4	6	6.5	7	7.5
General Hospital—Psych	4.8	4	3	4	4	5	5.5	6	6.5
General Hospital—Rehab	6.2	6	5	6	6	6.5	6.5	7	7.5
General Hospital—Other	6	6	4.5	5.5	6	6	6.5	7	7.5
Pediatric Hospital	5.6	6	4	5	5	6	6	6.5	7
Psychiatric Hospital	4.5	4	3	4	4	4.5	5	5.5	6
Outpatient Clinic	6.2	6	4.5	5.5	6	6.5	7	7	8
Rehabilitation Center/Hospital	6.2	6	5	5.5	6	6	6.7	7	7.5
School System	5.4	5	4	5	5	5.5	6	6	6.5
Skilled Nursing Facility/ICF	5.8	6	4.5	5	5.5	6	6	6.5	7
Sheltered Workshop	5.2	5.5	2.5	5	5	5.5	6	6	6.5
Vocational/Prevocational Program	6	6	4.6	5.5	5.8	6	6.2	6.5	7

Source: 1990 AOTA Member Data Survey

Table 3.13 Hours per day in direct patient service by primary work setting for COTAs employed full-time in direct patient service.

Setting	Mean	Mode	Percentiles						
			10	25	33.3	50	66.6	75	90
Community Mental Health Center	5.4	5	4	5	5	5.5	6	6.1	7.1
Day Care Program	5.7	6	4	5.3	5.5	6	6.3	6.5	7.3
Home Health Agency	6.3	6	2.6	5.5	6	6	6.8	7.5	10.2
General Hospital—Psych	5.4	5.5	3.5	4.5	5.2	5.5	6	6.5	7.2
General Hospital—Rehab	6.5	7.5	5.5	6	6	6.5	7	7	7.5
General Hospital—Other	5.9	6	4.5	5.5	5.5	6	6.5	7	7.5
Pediatric Hospital	6.1	6.5	—	5.3	6	6.5	6.5	7.3	—
Psychiatric Hospital	5.1	5	3.5	4	4.5	5	5.5	6	6.5
Outpatient Clinic	6.4	6.5	5	5.8	6	6.5	7	7	8
Rehabilitation Center/Hospital	6.5	7	5	6	6	6.5	7	7.1	8
School System	5.5	6	4	5	5	5.5	6	6.5	7
Skilled Nursing Facility/ICF	5.9	6	4.5	5.2	5.5	6	6.5	6.9	7.5
Sheltered Workshop	5.5	6	3.3	5	5.3	6	6	6.2	6.8
Vocational/Prevocational Program	6	6	4.8	5.5	5.6	6	6.3	6.5	7.4

Source: 1990 AOTA Member Data Survey

Managing Productivity in Occupational Therapy

Table 3.14 Hours per day in direct patient service by primary work setting for OTRs employed full-time as administrators.

Setting	Mean	Mode	Percentiles						
			10	25	33.3	50	66.6	75	90
Community Mental Health Center	2.2	1	0.9	1	1	2	3	3	4.4
Home Health Agency	3.3	3.5	0.9	1.5	1.8	3.5	4	4.4	7.3
General Hospital—Psych	2.7	1	1	1.5	2	2.5	3.5	3.6	4.7
General Hospital—Rehab	3.5	4	1	2	2	3.5	4	4.9	6.2
General Hospital—Other	3.6	3	1	2	2.5	3.5	4.5	5	6.5
Pediatric Hospital	2.8	3	1	2	2	2.5	3	3.5	5
Psychiatric Hospital	2.4	2	0.7	1	1.5	2	3	3	4.6
Outpatient Clinic	3.8	1	0.6	1.1	2	4	5.3	5.9	7.9
Rehabilitation Center/Hospital	3.2	2	1	1.5	2	2.5	4	4.5	6.5
School System	3.6	2	1.4	2	2.3	3.5	4	5.3	6
Skilled Nursing Facility/ICF	3.6	4	1	2	2.5	3.5	4.8	5	6.4
Sheltered Workshop	2.9	1	0.6	1	1.3	2.5	4	4.4	6

Source: 1990 AOTA Member Data Survey

Table 3.15 Hours per day in direct patient service by primary work setting for OTRs employed full-time as supervisors.

Setting	Mean	Mode	Percentiles						
			10	25	33.3	50	66.6	75	90
Home Health Agency	2.7	1	0.6	1	1	1.5	4	4.5	6.2
General Hospital—Psych	3.4	4	1.3	2.5	2.5	3.5	4	4	6
General Hospital—Rehab	4	6	1.5	2.5	3	4	5	6	6.5
General Hospital—Other	3.9	4	1.7	2.5	3	4	4.5	5	6
Pediatric Hospital	3.7	2	2	2.6	3.1	3.5	4.3	4.9	5.5
Psychiatric Hospital	2.5	2	1	1.5	2	2	3	3.6	4
Outpatient Clinic	4.2	4	1.2	2.7	3.6	4.3	5.1	5.5	6.5
Rehabilitation Center/Hospital	3.8	4	1.5	2.3	3	4	4.5	5	6.5
School System	3.3	2.5	1	2	2.5	3	4	4.6	5.7
Skilled Nursing Facility/ICF	4.1	3.5	1.7	3	3.5	4	5	5.5	6.5

Source: 1990 AOTA Member Data Survey

Table 3.16 Hours per day in direct patient service by primary work setting for OTRs employed full-time as consultants.

Setting	Mean	Mode	Percentiles						
			10	25	33.3	50	66.6	75	90
General Hospital—Other	5.6	6.5	3.7	5	5	5.5	6.5	6.5	7.1
Psychiatric Hospital	3.9	4	1.6	2.4	3.2	4	4	4.5	7.4
Rehabilitation Center/Hospital	5.5	4	3.3	4	4	5	6.8	7	7.7
School System	4.5	5	2	4	4	5	5.5	5.5	6.5
Skilled Nursing Facility/ICF	4	4	2	2.6	3	4	4.9	5	6

Source: 1990 AOTA Member Data Survey

Managing Productivity in Occupational Therapy

Appendices

This section contains a variety of selections that complete and supplement the materials presented earlier.

Appendix A is the questionnaire that was sent to contributors to this book in order to compile the facts presented in Section 2.

Appendix B was also sent to the contributors to give them a precise guide to the classification of occupational therapy personnel. The definitions presented in Appendix B are used throughout this book.

Appendix C presents a Summary Report of AOTA's 1990 Member Data Survey. This material supplements the data presented in Section 3.

Appendix D presents a list of recommended readings in the area covered by this book.

Finally, **Appendix E** provides the names and addresses of two organizations that can provide additional information on productivity.

PRODUCTIVITY QUESTIONNAIRE

Name:_____Title:_____

Facility:_____Address:_____

_____Phone (w):(   )_____

City   State   Zip

I. SETTINGS: Check all settings for which you will be supplying productivity information. Do not combine information from more than one setting on page 3. <u>For each setting checked below, please complete a separate page 3.</u>

[ ] Acute Mental Health Unit in General Hospital

[ ] Community Mental Health

[ ] Day Care Program

[ ] General Hospital *(NICU)*

[ ] General Hospital *(Rehab)*

[ ] General Hospital *(all other)*

[ ] Group Home or Independent Living Center

[ ] HMO/PPO/IPA

[ ] Home Health Agency

[ ] Hospice

[ ] Outpatient Clinic *(freestanding)*

[ ] Outpatient Clinic *(connected to a General Hospital)*

[ ] Partial Hospitals

[ ] Pediatric Hospital

[ ] Physician's Office

[ ] Private Industry

[ ] Private Practice

[ ] Psychiatric Hospital

[ ] Public Health Agency

[ ] Rehabilitation Agency

[ ] Rehabilitation Hospital

[ ] Residential Care Facility

[ ] Retirement or Senior Center

[ ] School System *(including private)*

[ ] Sheltered Workshop. Transitional Program, Supported Employment

[ ] Skilled Nursing Facility in General Hospital

[ ] Skilled Nursing Facility or Intermediate Care Facility
    [ ] Private   [ ] Public

[ ] Voluntary Agency *(UCP, Easter Seal)*

[ ] Work Hardening

[ ] Other_____
              specify

_____

II.A. Which of the following are considered as "direct billable time" or "direct patient service" at your setting? *(Check all that apply.)*

[ ] hands-on treatment

[ ] preparation time

[ ] treatment planning

[ ] charting

[ ] note writing

[ ] team meetings

[ ] family conferences

[ ] Other_____
              specify

B. As part of your productivity system, do you keep track of "nonbillable time," e.g., inservices, chart reviews, rounds? *(Check one.)* [ ] YES   [ ] NO

C. Which of the following units do you use for billing or recording productivity? *(Check all that apply.)*

    [ ] units of time

    [ ] RVUs *(relative value units)*

    [ ] procedures

    [ ] visits

    [ ] combination of above

    [ ] other:_____
                 specify

D. If you use units of time, which unit is most often used? *(Check one only.)*

    [ ] 10 minute units   [ ] 30 minute units

    [ ] 15 minute units   [ ] other:_____
                                         specify

E. When conducting staff evaluations/performance appraisals, are productivity measures used as part of the evaluation criteria? *(Check one.)* [ ] YES   [ ] NO

> **FOR EACH SETTING CHECKED ON PAGE 1, PART I INDICATE THE TYPE OF SETTING BELOW AND COMPLETE A SEPARATE FORM FOR EACH. DUPLICATE THIS FORM AS NEEDED.**

III. TYPE OF SETTING:_____

    A. Number of beds *(if applicable).* _____beds

    B. Total number of FTEs* for this setting. _____FTEs

    C. What is the productivity standard (in hours) for each of the following staff positions in direct patient/client service/billable time? **NOTE: REFER TO THE ENCLOSED "GUIDE TO CLASSIFICATION OF OCCUPATIONAL THERAPY PERSONNEL" FOR DEFINITIONS OF THE CATEGORIES BELOW.** *(If not applicable, leave blank.)*

OTR ENTRY LEVEL _____ hrs   COTA ENTRY LEVEL _____ hrs

OTR INTERMEDIATE LEVEL _____ hrs   COTA INTERMEDIATE LEVEL _____ hrs

OTR ADVANCED LEVEL _____ hrs   COTA ADVANCED LEVEL _____ hrs

        MANAGER/DIRECTOR ____ hrs

        FIELDWORK SUPERVISOR/COORDINATOR _____ hrs

        OT AIDE ____ hrs

        OTHER _____ _____ hrs
              specify

You may use the back of this form for any comments or explanations necessary. Thank you for completing this survey(s). Please return by **March 29, 1991** *to:*

PRACTICE DIVISION
THE AMERICAN OCCUPATIONAL THERAPY ASSOCIATION, INC.
PO BOX 1725
ROCKVILLE MD 20849-1725

* Full-Time Equivalent OT Staff

Guide to Classification of Occupational Therapy Personnel

The Guide to Classification of Occupational Therapy Personnel has been developed as a resource for the American Occupational Therapy Association, and for health care administrators and others requiring the services of occupational therapy personnel. The guide to common job roles of occupational therapy describes the qualifications and performance expectations of associated roles. The job roles are referred to as classifications; the classifications addressed are (a) staff occupational therapist, registered (OTR), including entry level, intermediate, and advanced; (b) staff certified occupational therapy assistant (COTA), including entry level, intermediate, and advanced; (c) occupational therapy supervisor; and (d) occupational therapy department manager/director.

This listing represents roles found typically in departments of institutions and is *not* intended to address the other roles occupational therapists perform in health care and educational settings. Other roles not addressed include, but are not limited to, private practitioner, consultant, faculty member, researcher, clinical coordinator, and administrator of multiservice departments.

The document describes performance areas that assist in definition of job roles and responsibilities of various occupational therapy personnel. The levels of personnel were chosen to reflect advancement with those who provide direct treatment services. The terms *intermediate* and *advanced* were specifically selected to reflect the degree of clinical expertise rather than longevity within the profession. The levels of management personnel (supervisor, department manager/director) also were chosen to reflect advancement in administrative roles.

Description of Personnel Classifications

Each description is organized in outline form, and includes the following components:

1. Suggested job title;

2. Primary Function: A brief description of the job; and

3. Qualifications: The necessary and preferred requirements for persons employed in this classification.

A. Education: Minimum and preferred educational preparation necessary to perform the job.

B. Certification and licensure: Statement of professional and legal credentials required. (Exceptions to these qualifications may occur in the case of newly graduated entry-level personnel. In states that license occupational therapy personnel, temporary provisions within the state law delineate requirements.)

C. Experience: Minimum and preferred experience necessary to perform the job adequately.

D. Skills: Description of minimum and preferred skills required to perform the job adequately.

4. Examples of Critical Performance Areas: Statements of the duties and responsibilities typical of the job classification. This listing is not comprehensive. Examples have been provided that reflect the level of competence and degree of independence expected in the performance of various job components.

- Indicates basic critical performance areas.

○ Indicates performance areas at higher levels.

5. Supervisory Support Needed: Description of both minimum and preferred supervision necessary for job performance. CLINICAL refers to supervision related to patient's/client's treatment. MANAGEMENT/ADMINISTRATIVE refers to supervision related to general duties of a nontreatment nature.

Additional Resources

The American Occupational Therapy Association (AOTA) has a variety of resources to assist members, groups, and other interested individuals in the development and implementation of occupational therapy programs and services. These resources include documents related to roles and functions of occupational therapy in various areas of practice, entry level role delineation of OTR/COTA personnel, standards of practice, and ethics. Information regarding reimbursement of services may be obtained from the AOTA, state occupational therapy associations, state and federal regulatory agencies, and private insurers. To obtain AOTA resource information and listings of state occupational therapy associations, contact The American Occupational Therapy Association, Inc., 1383 Piccard Drive, Suite 300, Rockville, MD 20850, (301)948-9626.

Occupational Therapy Personnel Classifications

Staff Occupational Therapist, Registered (OTR) Entry Level

Primary Function

To provide occupational therapy services to patients/clients, including assessment, treatment program planning and implementation, related documentation, and communication.

Qualifications

(All points must be met.)

1. *Certification:* By the American Occupational Therapy Certification Board (AOTCB) or satisfaction of any current state legal requirements; and

2. *Experience:* Less than one year as an OTR; and

3. *Skills:* Professional competency as a general practitioner of occupational therapy, as defined by AOTA.

Examples of Critical Performance Areas

• Responds to requests for service and initiates referrals where appropriate.

• Screens individuals to determine need for intervention.

• Evaluates patients/clients to obtain and interpret data necessary for treatment planning and implementation.

• Interprets evaluation findings to patients/clients, family, significant others, and care team.

• Develops treatment plans, including goals and methods to achieve identified goals.

• Coordinates treatment plan with patients/clients, family, significant others, and care team.

• Implements treatment directly or supervises treatment by a certified occupational therapy assistant.

• Monitors patient's/client's response to intervention and modifies treatment as indicated to attain goals.

• Develops appropriate home or community programming to maintain and enhance the performance of the patients/clients in their own environments.

• Terminates services when maximum benefit has been achieved.

• Documents results of patient's/client's assessment, treatment, follow-up, and termination of services.

• Reviews the quality and appropriateness of the total services delivered and of individual occupational therapy programs for effectiveness and efficiency, using predetermined criteria.

• Maintains service-related records.

• Follows billing and reimbursement procedures.

• Provides inservice education to members of the patient's/client's care team and education to the community.

• Complies with established agency standards and evaluates compliance.

• Identifies own continuing education and consultation needs.

• Supervises COTAs, occupational therapy aides and volunteers.

• Supervises occupational therapy and occupational therapy assistant Level I Fieldwork students.

Supervisory Support Needed

1. *Clinical:* Close supervision (i.e., daily direct contact on-site) from an intermediate or advanced level OTR is preferred. If not provided, general supervision (i.e., less than daily) or consultation, or both, by an intermediate or advanced level therapist is recommended. Frequency and manner of contact is determined by the supervising OTR, with on-site contact occurring at least monthly. Therapists may require consultation by an advanced level OTR in special areas in which they have minimal experience.

2. *Management/Administrative:* Administrative supervision is recommended for implementation of policies, quality assurance, and materiel management. In addition, supervision, or consultation, or both, by an OTR with administrative experience is recommended in the development of service operations, policies, and procedures related to billing, reimbursement, and adherence to state and federal regulatory requirements.

Staff Occupational Therapist, Registered (OTR) Intermediate Level

Primary Function

To provide occupational therapy services to patients/clients, including assessment, treatment program planning and implementation, related documentation, and communication.

Qualifications

(All points must be met.)

1. *Certification:* By the American Occupational Therapy Certification Board (AOTCB) or satisfaction of any current state legal requirements; and

2. *Experience:* One or more years of practice as an OTR; and

3. *Skills:* Professional competency as a general practitioner of occupational therapy as defined by AOTA.

Examples of Critical Performance Areas

• Indicates basic critical performance areas.
○ Indicates performance areas at higher levels.

• Responds to requests for service and initiates referrals when appropriate.

• Screens individuals to determine need for intervention.

• Evaluates patients/clients to obtain and interpret data necessary for treatment planning and implementation.

• Interprets evaluation findings to patients/clients, family, significant others, and care team.

• Develops treatment plans, including goals and methods to achieve identified goals.

• Coordinates treatment plan with patients/clients, family, significant others, and care team.

• Implements treatment directly or supervises treatment by a certified occupational therapy assistant.

• Monitors patient's/client's response to intervention and modifies treatment as indicated to attain goals.

• Develops appropriate home or community programming to maintain and enhance the performance of the patients/clients in their own environment.

• Terminates services when benefit has been achieved.

• Documents results of patient's/client's evaluation, treatment, follow-up, and termination of services.

• Identifies own continuing education and consultation needs.

• Follows billing and reimbursement procedures.

• Complies with established agency standards and evaluates compliance.

○ Maintains service-related records and assists in development of records.

○ Develops and provides inservice education to members of the patient's/client's care team and to the community.

○ Reviews the quality and appropriateness of the total services delivered and of individual occupational therapy programs for effectiveness and efficiency, using predetermined criteria.

○ Develops treatment protocols and procedures for patient's/client's programs within scope of own experience.

○ Supervises COTAs, occupational therapy aides, and volunteers.

○ Supervises occupational therapy and occupational therapy assistant Level I and II Fieldwork students.

○ Participates in the development of service operations, policies, and procedures.

Supervisory Support Needed

1. *Clinical:* General supervision (i.e., less than daily) by a more experienced intermediate or advanced level OTR is preferred for therapists with less than two years' experience. Frequency and manner of contact is determined by the supervising OTR, with on-site contact occurring at least monthly. Therapists may require consultation by an advanced level OTR in special areas in which they have minimal experience.

2. *Management/Administrative:* Administrative supervision is required for implementation of policies, quality assurance, and materiel management. In addition, supervision or consultation, or both, by an OTR with administrative experience is required in the development of service operations, policies, and procedures related to billing, reimbursement, and adherence to state and federal regulatory requirements.

Staff Occupational Therapist, Registered (OTR) Advanced Level

An advanced level occupational therapist may function as a staff therapist, but at a level higher than an intermediate therapist. Because of the variety of ways an individual may obtain advanced-level skills and the variety of jobs that an individual may perform, specific qualifications and critical performance areas cannot be delineated. An advanced level therapist should be able to meet all the expectations in the personnel classification of **Staff OTR, Intermediate Level,** and should demonstrate the following education, experience, and skills.

Qualifications

(All points must be met.)

1. *Education:* Continuing education, examination, and/or practice requirements; and/or extensive continuing education in special area of practice is recommended; and

2. *Experience:* Three or more years of experience in special area of practice; and

3. *Skills:* An advanced level therapist has skills that reflect a range of experience and depth of knowledge in occupational therapy theory and practice. Integration of clinical theory and practice at the advanced level results in evaluation and treatment that is innovative, complex, and efficient. The advanced level therapist could be expected to share knowledge through staff and student education, publications, clinical studies, and research.

Examples of Critical Performance Areas

• Indicates basic critical performance areas.

○ Because of the variety of ways an individual may obtain advanced-level skills and the variety of jobs that an individual may perform, critical performance areas at higher levels cannot be delineated.

• Responds to requests for service and initiates referrals when appropriate.

• Screens individuals to determine need for intervention.

• Evaluates patients/clients to obtain and interpret data necessary for treatment planning and implementation.

• Interprets evaluation findings to patients/clients, family, significant others, and care team.

• Develops treatment plans, including goals and methods to achieve identified goals.

• Coordinates treatment plan with patients/clients, family, significant others, and care team.

• Implements treatment directly or supervises treatment by a certified occupational therapy assistant.

• Monitors patient's/client's response to intervention and modifies treatment as indicated to attain goals.

• Develops appropriate home or community programming to maintain and enhance the performance of the patients/clients in their own environment.

- Terminates services when benefit has been achieved.
- Documents results of patient's/client's evaluation, treatment, follow-up, and termination of services.
- Identifies own continuing education and consultation needs.
- Follows billing and reimbursement procedures.
- Maintains service-related records and assists in development of records.
- Develops and provides inservice education to members of the patient's/client's care team and to the community.
- Reviews the quality and appropriateness of the total services delivered and of individual occupational therapy programs for effectiveness and efficiency, using predetermined criteria.
- Develops treatment protocols and procedures for patient's/client's programs within scope of own experience.
- Supervises COTAs, occupational therapy aides, and volunteers.
- Supervises occupational therapy and occupational therapy assistant Level I and II Fieldwork students.
- Participates in the development of service operations, policies, and procedures.

Supervisory Support Needed

1. *Clinical:* General supervision as required. Supervision is not required when treating within an area of special practice. Occasional supervision and consultation may be needed in other areas.

2. *Management/Administrative:* Administrative supervision is recommended for implementation of policies, quality assurance, and materiel management. In addition, supervision or consultation, or both, by an OTR with administrative experience is recommended in the development of service operations, policies, and procedures related to billing, reimbursement, and adherence to state and federal regulatory requirements.

Staff Certified Occupational Therapy Assistant (COTA) Entry Level

Primary Function

To implement occupational therapy services for patients and clients under the supervision of an occupational therapist (OTR). These services include structured assessments, treatments, and documentation.

Qualifications

(All points must be met.)

1. *Certification:* By the American Occupational Therapy Certification Board (AOTCB) or satisfaction of any current state legal requirements; and

2. *Experience:* Less than one year of practice experience as a COTA; and

3. *Skills:* Competent in the delivery of occupational therapy treatment, under the direction of an OTR as delineated in the AOTA Entry-Role Delineation for OTRs and COTAs.

Examples of Critical Performance Areas

- Indicates basic critical performance areas.
- ○ Indicates performance areas at higher levels.

- Responds to requests for service by relaying information and referral to an OTR.
- Determines patient's/client's need for services in collaboration with an OTR.
- Contributes to the assessment process under supervision of an OTR.
- Assists OTR in developing treatment plans and techniques to implement plans.
- Monitors patient's/client's response to treatment and modifies treatment during sessions as indicated in collaboration with an OTR.
- Reports observations of patient's/client's performance and responses to services to the OTR.
- Recommends termination of patient/client services to the supervisor.
- Documents and maintains service-related records, as directed by supervising OTR.
- Assists in providing inservice education.
- Complies with established agency and service standards.
- Identifies own continuing education needs in consultation with OTR.

Supervisory Support Needed

1. *Clinical:* Close supervision (i.e., daily direct contact on-site) is required from an OTR or intermediate or advanced level COTA.

2. *Management/Administrative:* General supervision by an experienced OTR or an experienced COTA is required for implementation of policies and procedures related to delivery of occupational therapy services.

Staff Certified Occupational Therapy Assistant (COTA) Intermediate Level

Primary Function

To implement occupational therapy services for patients/clients under the supervision of an occupational therapist (OTR). These services include structured evaluations, treatment, and documentation.

Qualifications

(All points must be met.)

1. *Certification:* By the American Occupational Therapy Certification Board (AOTCB) or satisfaction of any current state legal requirements; and

2. *Experience:* One or more years of practice as a COTA; and

3. *Skills:* Competent in delivery of occupational therapy treatment under the direction of an OTR as delineated in the AOTA Entry-Level Role Delineation document; skill in implementation of a variety of independent living skills and activities that can be used in treatment; may be developing advanced-level skills in areas of special interest.

Examples of Critical Performance Areas

- Indicates basic critical performance areas.
- Indicates performance areas at higher levels.

- Responds to requests for service by relaying information and referral to an OTR.
- Determines patient's/client's need for services in collaboration with an OTR.
- Contributes to the patient's/client's assessment under supervision of an OTR. Independently performs parts of assessments, using structured evaluations.
- Assists OTR in developing treatment plans and techniques to implement plans.
- Implements and modifies treatment plans, under OTR supervision.
- Monitors patient's/client's response to treatment and modifies treatment during sessions, as indicated, in collaboration with OTR.
- Reports observations and patient's/client's responses to service to OTR and to other team members when so directed by OTR.
- Recommends to supervisor the termination of services.
- Documents and maintains service-related records, as directed by supervising OTR.
- Assists in the development of treatment protocols.
- Assists in the development of service records and procedures.
- Identifies own continuing education needs.
- Provides inservice education, and community education within scope of knowledge base.
- Provides administrative supervision and clinical direction to entry-level COTAs.
- Supervises OT aides and volunteers.
- Provides administration and clinical direction to OT Assistant Levels I and II Fieldwork students.
- Assists OTR in the implementation of quality assurance program.
- Complies with established agency and service standards.

Supervisory Support Needed

1. *Clinical:* General supervision (i.e. less than daily) from an intermediate or advanced level OTR is required. For COTAs with less than two years' experience, close supervision (i.e. daily direct contact on-site) is preferred.

The nature and frequency of supervision varies with patient/client populations. COTAs working with acutely ill patients/clients and with individuals who are making rapid changes will require more OTR supervision, due to the need for frequent evaluation and re-evaluation and the resulting modification of overall treatment plan. COTAs treating patients/clients whose conditions are less complex and more stable, and therefore require program revisions less frequently, may be directed by the OTR to function more independently. Frequency and manner of contact is determined by the supervising OTR with on-site contact occurring at least monthly.

2. *Management/Administrative:* General supervision by an OTR experienced in administration or an advanced level COTA is required for implementation of policies and procedures related to the delivery of occupational therapy services.

Staff Certified Occupational Therapy Assistant (COTA) Advanced Level

An advanced level certified occupational therapy assistant (COTA) may function as a staff member, but at a higher level than an intermediate COTA. Because of the variety of ways an individual may obtain advanced level skills and the variety of jobs that an individual may perform, specific qualifications and critical performance areas cannot be delineated. An advanced level COTA should be able to meet all the expectations of a **Staff COTA (Intermediate Level)** and the following education, experience, and skills.

Qualifications

(All points must be met.)

1. *Education:* Academic course work related to area of expertise from an accredited college or university; and/or certification related to a special area of practice by an organization or group that has continuing education, examination, and/or practice requirements; and/or extensive continuing education in special area of practice is recommended; and

2. *Experience:* Three years or more experience in special area of practice; and

3. *Skills:* A COTA in this category has advanced level competencies in particular acquired skills that relate to the practice of occupational therapy. These skills may be in clinically specific areas or may be more administrative or educational in nature. The advanced level COTA could be expected to share knowledge through staff and student education, publications, and clinical studies.

Examples of Critical Performance Areas

- Indicates basic critical performance areas.
- Because of the variety of ways an individual may obtain advanced level skills and the variety of jobs

an individual may perform, critical performance areas at higher levels cannot be delineated.

- Responds to requests for service by relaying information and referral to an OTR.
- Determines patient's/client's need for services in collaboration with an OTR.
- Contributes to the patient's/client's assessment under supervision of an OTR. Independently performs parts of assessments, using structured evaluations.
- Assists OTR in developing treatment plans and techniques to implement plans.
- Implements and modifies treatment plans, under OTR supervision.
- Monitors patient's/client's response to treatment and modifies treatment during sessions, as indicated, in collaboration with OTR.
- Reports observations and patient's/client's responses to service to OTR and to other team members when so directed by OTR.
- Recommends to supervisor the termination of services.
- Documents and maintains service-related records, as directed by supervising OTR.
- Assists in the development of treatment protocols.
- Assists in the development of service records and procedures.
- Identifies own continuing education needs.
- Provides inservice education, and community education within scope of knowledge base.
- Provides administrative supervision and clinical direction to entry-level COTAs.
- Supervises OT aides and volunteers.
- Provides administration and clinical direction to OT Assistant Levels I and II Fieldwork students.
- Assists OTR in the implementation of quality assurance program.
- Complies with established agency and service standards.

Supervisory Support Needed

1. *Clinical:* General supervision (i.e., less than daily) from an intermediate or advanced-level OTR is required. The nature and frequency of supervision varies with patient's/client's population. COTAs working with acutely ill patients and with individuals who are making rapid changes will require more OTR supervision, because of the need for frequent evaluation and re-evaluation and resulting modification of overall treatment plan. COTAs treating patients whose conditions are less complex and more stable, therefore require program revisions less frequently, may be directed by the OTR to function more independently.

2. *Management/Administrative:* General supervision by an administratively experienced OTR is required for implementation of service policies and procedures.

Occupational Therapy Supervisor

Primary Function

To supervise OTRs, COTAs, students, volunteers, and aides. Supervision includes orientation, development, and evaluation of personnel and monitoring of quality provision of services. Patient/client care responsibilities will vary depending on volume of personnel to be supervised. May serve as Fieldwork coordinator.

Qualifications

1. *Education:* Continuing education relevant to the supervisory function is recommended; and

2. *Certification:* By the American Occupational Therapy Certification Board (AOTCB) or satisfaction of any current state legal requirements; and

3. *Experience:* Three or more years of clinical experience that is related to the departmental scope of service provided; and

4. *Skills:* Thorough understanding of personnel and departmental policies and procedures; demonstrated leadership potential and ability to communicate effectively with peers, subordinates, and management; demonstrated ability to organize use of time, material, and personnel effectively; intermediate or advanced clinical skills.

Examples of Critical Performance Areas

- Indicates basic critical performance areas.
○ Indicates performance areas at higher levels.

- Assists in the selection and orientation of staff, students, and volunteers.
- Evaluates and monitors job performance of assigned staff.
- Coordinates and facilitates inservice education and professional development of assigned staff.
- Coordinates scheduling of work assignments.
- Implements departmental policies and procedures, identifies need for changes, and assists in development and revision.
- Develops, implements, and maintains quality assurance activities within assigned areas.
- Assists in identification and development of department goals and objectives.
- Develops and implements strategies to meet department goals and objectives under supervision of department manager.
- Coordinates student fieldwork education.
- Is knowledgeable of and monitors staff compliance with AOTA professional guidelines, standards, and ethics.
- Assists department manager in ensuring department compliance with relevant accreditation, certification, and government standards.
- Performs assigned patient/client care responsibilities.

Supervisory Support Needed

1. *Clinical:* General supervision by occupational therapy department or service manager/director is required. Consultation from advanced-level OTR is recommended for special areas of practice in which therapist has had minimal experience.

2. *Management/Administrative:* General supervision by occupational therapy department manager/director is required for assigned supervisory duties.

Occupational Therapy Department Manager/Director

Primary Function

To manage an occupational therapy department or service. Management includes planning, organizing, directing, controlling, and coordinating all aspects of the department or service.

Qualifications

1. *Education:* Continuing education relevant to the management/administrative function is recommended; and

2. *Certification:* By the American Occupational Therapy Certification Board (AOTCB) or satisfaction of any current state legal requirements; and

3. *Experience:* Varies with size and scope of department. Graduate degree in administration and management may substitute for supervisory experience.

    a. Small department (less than six employees): Three years or more clinical experience as an occupational therapist, with a minimum of one year of supervisory experience.

    b. Large department (more than six employees): Four or more years of clinical experience, with at least two years of supervisory and management experience; and

4. *Skills:* Intermediate or advanced-level clinical skills. Must have a thorough knowledge of occupational therapy and management principles and practices; demonstrate understanding of department objectives and functions; and conceptualize,, interpret, and integrate occupational therapy services into the relevant organizational context.

Examples of Critical Performance Areas

- • Indicates basic critical performance areas.
- ○ Indicates performance areas at higher levels.

- • Selects, evaluates, and maintains competent staff.
- • Develops, implements, and monitors policies and procedures within department.
- • Participates in interdepartmental development of systems, policies, and procedures. Identifies system dysfunctions and reports to appropriate administrative personnel.

- • Participates in development of organizational goals and plans and supports organizational objectives.
- • Establishes, coordinates, and maintains effective relationships with other departments, the administration, and the community.
- • Supports financial management of the organization through budget preparation and implementation, and reviews and develops related reports.
- • Identifies departmental program changes, and develops and implements strategies to provide relevant cost-effective services.
- • Develops and implements quality assurance and program evaluation systems within department.
- • Collaborates with other departments and administration in the development and implementation of interdepartmental evaluation systems.
- • Is knowledgeable of and ensures compliance with accreditation, certification, and government standards that are relevant to the department.
- • Is knowledgeable of and ensures compliance with AOTA professional guidelines, standards, and ethics.

Supervisory Support Needed

General supervision by administrative personnel within the organization is required.

Glossary of Terms

1. *Assessment*—Occupational therapy assessment refers to the process of determining the need for, nature of, and estimated time of treatment; determining the needed coordination with other persons involved; and documenting these activities (1).

2. *Evaluation*—Evaluation refers to the process of obtaining and interpreting data necessary for treatment (2). This includes planning for and documenting the evaluation process and results. These data may be gathered through record review, specific observation, interview, and the administration of data collection procedures. Such procedures include but are not limited to the use of standardized tests, performance checklists, and activities and tasks designed to evaluate specific performance abilities. The following categories of occupational therapy evaluation include independent living/daily living skills and performance, and their components:

    a. Independent Living/Daily Living Skills and Performance;

    b. Sensorimotor Skill and Performance Components;

    c. Cognitive Skill and Performance Components;

    d. Psychosocial Skill and Performance Components;

    e. Therapeutic Adaptations;

    f. Specialized Evaluations.

Specialized evaluations refer to evaluations or tests requiring specialized training and/or advanced education to administer and interpret them. Examples of specialized evaluations are employment preparation, prevocational testing, sensory integration, prosthetic, and driver training.

3. *Supervision*—Supervision refers to activities to enhance the performance of departmental employees through appraisal of their effectiveness, evaluation of their conformance to departmental standards, and/or evaluation of their adherence to specific institutional policies (2).

a. *Close*—requires daily, direct contact on-site.

b. *General*—in which frequency of contact is less than daily. Frequency and manner of contact is determined by the supervising OTR, with on-site contact occurring at least monthly. Interim supervision should occur in some manner (e.g., via telephone, written report, group conference).

REFERENCES

1. American Occupational Therapy Association (1979). *Uniform terminology for reporting occupational therapy product output reporting system.* Rockville, MD: Author.
2. American Occupational Therapy Association (1981). Guide for supervision of occupational therapy personnel. *American Journal of Occupational Therapy, 35*(12), 815–816. Rockville, MD: Author.

Author: Barbara A. Boyt Schell, MS, OTR/L
Contributors: Caroline R. Brayley, MEd, OTR/L, FAOTA
Margaret W. Heister, OTR/L
Barbara M. Smith, OTR/L
Martha W. Smyers, OTR/L

For: AOTA Commission on Practice, Esther Bell, MA, OTR, FAOTA, Chair

Approved by the Representative Assembly April 1985
Edited June 1987

Note: This document replaces *Minimal Occupational Therapy Classification Standards* (May 1970, revised January 1977).

Managing Productivity in Occupational Therapy

1990
Member Data Survey

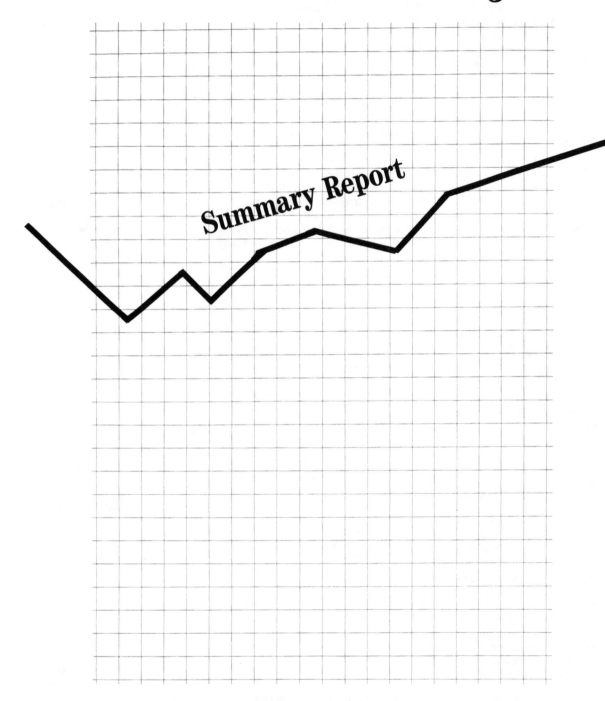

Summary Report

Research Information & Evaluation Division

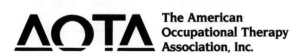 **The American Occupational Therapy Association, Inc.**   1383 Piccard Drive P.O. Box 1725
Rockville, MD 20850-0822
(301) 948-9626   (301) 948-5512 Fax

1990 MEMBER DATA SURVEY

Introduction

The American Occupational Therapy Association conducts a comprehensive census of its members every three-to-four years. The results of the survey are used to update member records, identify and follow trends in occupational therapy practice and education, plan for future needs of the profession, develop resource and mailing lists, and collect special data that is used by the Association for program planning and policy decisions. The data from the survey are also used to respond to thousands of requests for information from AOTA members and other individuals, federal, state and local governments.

The 1990 Member Data Survey was designed to gather updated information from members in the following areas: personal information, education history, present employment, and professional experience and needs in a variety of areas.

Survey Protocol

The questionnaire was mailed to each Registered Occupational Therapist (OTR) and Certified Occupational Therapy Assistant (COTA) in May, 1990. Portions of the survey form were preprinted with data about the respondent from the AOTA membership files. Respondents were asked to correct or update the existing permanent information. These categories of information included birth year, sex, ethnic origin and education.

Of the more than 40,000 surveys mailed, about 0.3% were found to be undeliverable by the post office. Some 20,000 surveys were completed and returned to the National Office. Each survey was edited and keypunched on tape for data entry. Permanent data on the individual from the AOTA Membership files (such as sex, ethnic origin, state of residence, education, age, etc.) were appended to the survey tape.

This summary report describes the percentages of responses to most survey items with annotations where warranted. More detailed information including numbers of non-responders per item, analyses of cross tabulations, trends and subsets of the data are available from the AOTA Research Information & Evaluation Division. In addition, an analysis of the representativeness of the survey data is planned. This analysis will compare demographically the responders to those who did not respond to the survey.

The survey also collected information on hourly wages, daily and half-daily rates for service and charges for various types of service. These data will be the subject of future articles in *OT Week*.

Data Usage

The percents contained in this report, with the exception of the demographic and educational information, represent only those individuals who responded to the Member Data Survey, unless noted otherwise. They do not include the occupational therapy personnel who chose not to answer and return the survey.

If one wished to report numbers rather than percents, the percentages indicated in this report should be multiplied by the appropriate count of occupational therapy personnel, for example, the number of OTs in the U.S. (38,900 OTRs or 9,500 COTAs) or the number of COTAs in Maryland (available from the Research Division). This procedure will yield reasonable approximations assuming that the survey results are representative. If you have any questions, please call the Research Information & Evaluation Division at 301-948-9626 or for AOTA members 1-800-SAY-AOTA.

Summary of Results

- A growing proportion of OT practitioners are employed (either full- or part-time), probably the result of the national economy and the severe shortages of personnel.

- The proportion of practitioners working primarily with mental health problems continues to decline.

- More occupational therapists and occupational therapy assistants are becoming self-employed or entering private practice.

- COTA employment in school systems continues to rise; OTRs rebound to the same proportion as ten years ago.

- Occupational therapists are working more often with patients who have back injuries, developmental delay, and learning disabilities; less often with cerebral palsy and arteriosclerosis.

- Salaries for OTRs and COTAs are increasing at an average of 8 percent annually. Salaries of new graduates have risen an average of 9 percent per year since 1986.

- Employment has grown in private profit-making institutions.

- Occupational therapists are less likely to be certified or licensed in other fields than they were in the past.

- OTRs are more likely to be employed in urban areas; the proportion of COTAs is greater in rural areas.

- COTAs are twice as likely as OTRs to be employed in fields other than occupational therapy.

- More than half of OTRs consider themselves "specialists" rather than "generalists."

- About a third of OTRs and a quarter of COTAs consider "consultation" to be their secondary employment function.

- COTAs are more likely to be working with the elderly; the proportion of OTRs is higher in pediatrics.

1990 MEMBER DATA SURVEY

Demographic Information

TABLE 1: Sex

Sex	OTRs %	COTAs %
Female	94.3	91.8
Male	5.7	8.2
Total	100.0	100.0

TABLE 2: Age

Age	OTRs %	COTAs %
20 thru 29 years	20.5	23.7
30 thru 39 years	45.5	48.1
40 thru 49 years	18.6	16.7
50 thru 59 years	8.2	5.9
60 thru 69 years	5.4	3.7
70+ years	1.8	1.7
Total	100.0	99.8

Median Age	36 years	33 years

TABLE 3: Ethnic Origin

Ethnic Origin	OTRs %	COTAs %
American Indian, Aluet or Eskimo	0.2	0.4
Asian or Pacific islander	3.1	0.9
Black	2.7	5.8
Hispanic	1.7	2.0
White	91.5	90.2
Other	0.8	0.7
Total	100.0	100.0

TABLE 4: Disabling Condition

Response	OTRs %	COTAs %
No	95.8	93.7
Yes	4.2	6.3
Total	100.0	100.0

Education Information

TABLE 5: Entry-Level OT Educational Degree

Degree	OTRs %	COTAs %
Diploma/Certificate	8.9	24.0
Associate	2.5	70.8
Baccalaureate	82.3	5.2
Masters	6.3	—
Total	100.0	100.0

TABLE 6: Highest-Level OT Educational Degree

Degree	OTRs %	COTAs %
Diploma/Certificate	8.0	25.2
Associate	0.5	73.8
Baccalaureate	80.8	0.9
Masters	10.7	0.1
Doctorate	0.0	0.0
Total	100.1	100.0

TABLE 7: Highest-Level Educational Degree*

Degree	OTRs %	COTAs %
Diploma/Certificate	2.6	21.7
Associate	0.8	70.7
Baccalaureate	78.8	6.8
Masters	17.0	0.7
Doctorate	0.8	0.0
Total	100.0	99.9

*in any field, including occupational therapy

TABLE 8: Other Licenses or Certifications

Fields	OTRs %	COTAs %
Education	4.3	2.2
Nursing	0.5	2.1
Physical Therapy	0.5	0.2
Psychology	0.3	0.3
Social Work	0.4	0.5
Special Education	1.9	0.7
Speech Pathology/Audiology	0.1	0.1
Therapeutic Recreation	0.3	1.1
Vocational Rehabilitation	0.5	0.2
Sensory Integration	5.9	0.4
Vocational Evaluation Specialist (CVE)	0.6	0.1
Work Adjustment Specialist (CWA)	0.2	0.1
Neurodevelopmental Treatment (NDT)	7.0	0.4
Other	3.4	4.5

TABLE 9: Degree Currently Being Pursued

Degree	OTRs %	COTAs %
Baccalaureate	4.2	85.0
Master's	78.2	15.0
Doctorate	16.6	0
Post-Doctorate	1.0	0
Total	100.0	100.0

Note: Approximately 10 percent of OTRs and 20 percent of COTAs are pursuing additional educational degrees.

Employment Information

TABLE 10: Control or Ownership of Employment Setting

Description	OTRs %	COTAs %
Federal, Vet. Admin.	2.1	0.9
Federal, Military	0.7	1.5
Federal, Other	0.5	0.5
State	13.6	15.9
City/County	17.5	18.2
Private, Profit	27.8	27.6
Private, Nonprofit	36.2	34.0
Other	1.5	1.5
Total	100.0	100.0

Note: Data based on primary employment setting. Comparable data for secondary employment settings are available.

TABLE 11: Job Changes in Past 2 Years

Changes	OTRs %	COTAs %
Zero	69.7	69.6
Once	23.4	21.8
Twice	5.2	5.8
Three times	1.4	2.4
Four times	0.2	0.3
Five or more times	0.1	0.0
Total	100.0	99.9

TABLE 12: Employed in Field other than OT

Response	OTRs %	COTAs %
No	90.4	81.4
Yes	9.6	18.6
Total	100.0	100.0

TABLE 13: Location of Worksite

Location	OTRs %	COTAs %
Urban	44.6	35.8
Suburban	40.4	39.6
Rural	15.0	24.5
Total	100.0	100.0

TABLE 14: Supply and/or Equipment Responsibility for Department

Response	OTRs %	COTAs %
No	34.6	49.5
Yes	65.4	50.5
Total	100.0	100.0

TABLE 15: AOTA Dues Paid by Employer

Response	OTRs %	COTAs %
No	87.0	88.0
Yes	13.0	12.0
Total	100.0	100.0

TABLE 16: Employment Status by Year - OTRs

	OTRs				
Employment Status	1973 %	1977 %	1982 %	1986 %	1990 %
Employed - Full-time	57.1	64.4	70.4	69.4	70.5
Employed - Part-time	14.3	14.6	16.7	18.9	20.3
Volunteer	1.4	1.1	0.6	0.4	0.4
Not Employed - plan to work	22.8	17.0	9.5	8.2	6.0
Not Employed - don't plan to work	4.4	2.7	2.8	3.1	2.8
Total	100.0	100.0	100.1	100.0	100.0

TABLE 17: Primary Employment Setting by Year

	OTRs				
Setting	1973	1977	1982	1986	1990
College, 2 yr.	1.4	1.2	0.8	0.7	0.6
College/Univ., 4 yr.	5.6	4.9	4.1	3.1	3.4
Comm. Mental Health Ctr.	4.2	4.3	2.4	1.6	1.1
Correctional Institution	0.2	0.2	0.1	0.1	—
Day Care Ctr./Program	1.4	1.1	1.0	1.1	0.9
HMO (incl. PPO/IPA)	0.3	0.2	0.2	0.3	0.4
Home Health Agency	0.9	2.2	3.8	4.6	3.6
Hospice	—	—	0.0	0.1	0.0
Gen. Hospital - Neonatal Intensive Care Unit	—	—	—	—	0.7
Gen. Hospital - Psych Unit	—	—	—	—	3.5
Gen. Hospital - Rehab. Unit	—	—	—	4.2	5.3
Gen. Hospital - all other	20.5	19.8	25.3	22.0	15.9
Pediatric Hospital	2.9	2.0	1.6	1.7	1.7
Psychiatric Hospital	13.8	11.2	7.4	6.9	4.6
Outpatient Clinic (free stdg.)	—	—	2.5	2.4	3.7
Physician's Office	—	—	—	1.1	1.2
Private Industry	—	—	0.7	0.5	0.8
Private Practice	1.3	2.1	3.5	6.0	7.7
Public Health Agency	1.6	1.5	0.8	0.9	0.9
Rehab. Hospital/Center	13.4	10.9	8.9	10.5	11.4
Research Facility	0.3	0.3	0.4	0.2	0.2
Residential Care Fac. incl. Group Home, Ind. Liv. Ctr.	—	4.4	4.2	3.3	2.7
Retirement or Senior Ctr.	—	—	—	0.2	0.2
School System (includes private school)	11.0	14.0	18.3	17.0	18.6
Sheltered Workshop	0.7	0.7	0.7	0.4	0.4
Skilled Nursing Home/ Int. Care Facility	6.2	7.9	6.0	5.8	6.4
Vocational or Prevoc. Prog.	0.7	0.5			
Voluntary Agency (eg, Easter Seal/U.C.P.)	—	1.7	1.7	1.4	1.0
Other	14.2	9.4	5.4	3.2	2.5
Total	99.9%	100.0%	99.8%	100.0%	99.9%

NOTE: Missing data are due to changing employment categories on the various administrations of the surveys. Recoding of additional settings in the "other" category into existing alternatives may explain the decline in the "other" category. For this reason, small differences in the percentages over time should be interpreted with care.

Employment Information

TABLE 18: Employment Status by Year - COTAs

Employment Status	COTAs				
	1973 %	1977 %	1982 %	1986 %	1990 %
Employed - Full-time	71.0	72.2	72.7	69.7	72.2
Employed - Part-time	6.2	6.9	11.0	14.5	17.0
Volunteer	1.3	1.0	1.1	0.5	0.6
Not Employed - plan to work	20.3	18.7	13.7	14.4	9.0
Not Employed - don't plan to work	1.2	1.2	1.5	1.0	1.2
Total	100.0	100.0	100.0	100.0	100.0

Setting	COTAs				
	1973	1977	1982	1986	1990
College, 2 yr.	0.8	0.9	0.6	0.8	0.9
College/Univ., 4 yr.	0.7	0.6	0.9	0.3	0.3
Comm. Mental Health Ctr.	4.0	3.5	3.1	3.8	1.7
Correctional Institution	0.3	0.2	0.1	0.2	–
Day Care Ctr./Program	1.2	2.4	2.0	4.3	1.7
HMO (incl. PPO/IPA)	0.7	0.3	0.3	0.2	0.1
Home Health Agency	0.2	0.4	0.8	1.2	1.5
Hospice	–	–	0.0	0.0	0.0
Gen. Hospital - Neonatal Intensive Care Unit	–	–	–	–	0.1
Gen. Hospital - Psych Unit	–	–	–	–	4.0
Gen. Hospital - Rehab. Unit	–	–	–	4.5	5.5
Gen. Hospital - all other	15.1	12.7	17.8	14.1	9.4
Pediatric Hospital	1.5	1.2	0.8	0.4	0.7
Psychiatric Hospital	22.6	14.3	9.7	8.4	6.6
Outpatient Clinic (free stdg.)	–	–	1.7	0.9	2.2
Physician's Office	–	–	–	0.2	0.3
Private Industry	1.0	0.5	0.7		
Private Practice	0.3	0.4	1.2	1.9	2.7
Public Health Agency	0.5	0.5	0.3	0.4	0.6
Rehab. Hospital/Center	9.5	11.0	8.4	8.4	10.9
Research Facility	0.2	0.3	0.1	0.0	0.2
Residential Care Fac. incl. Group Home, Ind. Liv. Ctr.	–	8.5	7.6	7.5	5.9
Retirement or Senior Ctr.	–	–	–	1.1	0.8
School System (includes private school)	3.6	6.2	11.3	14.4	17.0
Sheltered Workshop	1.4	0.9	1.9	1.6	1.6
Skilled Nursing Home/ Int. Care Facility	22.8	26.1	22.5	20.1	20.1
Vocational or Prevoc. Prog.	–	–	–	1.6	0.8
Voluntary Agency (eg, Easter Seal/U.C.P.)	–	0.4	1.2	1.2	1.1
Other	14.7	9.3	6.7	2.3	2.3
Total	100.1%	100.1%	100.0%	100.0%	99.8%

TABLE 19: Role in Occupational Therapy

Role	OTRs %	COTAs %
Generalist	41.8	61.2
Specialist	58.2	38.8
Total	100.0	100.0

TABLE 20: Serve on an Ethics Committee at Work

Response	OTRs %	COTAs %
No	96.6	97.3
Yes	3.4	2.7
Total	100.0	100.0

TABLE 21: Received Public Recognition for Work in Occupational Therapy

Response	OTRs %	COTAs %
No	77.8	87.2
Yes	22.2	12.8
Total	100.0	100.0

TABLE 22A: Daily Hours in Direct Patient/ Client Service*

Hours	OTRs	COTAs
Mean (1)	5.8	5.9
Median (2)	6.0	6.0
Mode (3)	6.0	6.0

TABLE 22B: Patients/Clients Seen Daily*

Patients	OTRs	COTAs
Mean (1)	9.3	10.8
Median (2)	8.0	9.0
Mode (3)	8.0	10.0

*Data represents responses from full-time occupational therapy personnel whose primary employment function is direct patient/client service
(1) Arithmetic Average
(2) Middle case (50 percentile)
(3) Most frequent answer

TABLE 23: Computer Usage in OT Practice

	OTRs %	COTAs %
For administration	48.3	30.3
For treatment	40.7	31.1

Employment Information

TABLE 24: Most Frequent Health Problems of Patients/Clients

Health Problems	OTRs %	COTAs %
Alzheimer's Disease	0.6	2.2
Amputation	0.1	0.3
Arteriosclerosis	0.1	0.3
Arthritis/Collagen Disorder	0.9	1.0
Back Injury	3.4	3.0
Burns	0.4	0.1
Cancer (Neoplasms)	0.2	0.3
Cardiopulmonary Diseases	0.7	0.4
Cerebral Palsy	9.7	6.0
Congenital Anomalies	0.3	0.1
CVA/Hemiplegia	27.1	30.3
Developmental Delay	12.9	8.9
Diabetes	0.1	0.1
Feeding Disorders	0.3	0.0
Fracture	2.3	3.0
Hand Injury	9.5	3.2
Hearing Disability	0.1	0.3
HIV Infections, incl. AIDS	0.1	0.0
Kidney Disorder	0.0	0.0
Learning Disabilities	7.0	5.1
Neuro/Muscular Disorder (e.g. MD, MS)	0.6	0.6
Respiratory Disease	0.1	0.2
Spinal Cord Injury	1.2	1.2
Traumatic Brain Injury	4.2	3.9
Visual Disability	0.3	0.0
Well Population	0.2	0.5
Adjustment Disorders	0.8	1.2
Affective Disorders	3.7	2.5
Alcohol/Substance Use Disorders	0.8	1.5
Anxiety Disorders	0.1	0.4
Eating Disorders	0.2	0.1
Mental Retardation	4.9	11.4
Organic Mental Disorders*	0.8	2.1
Personality Disorders	0.6	0.8
Schizophrenic Disorders	4.1	6.6
Other Psychotic Disorders	0.1	0.2
Other Mental Health Disorders	0.6	1.1
Other:_____	0.8	1.1
Total	100.0	100.0

* Including Dementias and Organic Brain Syndromes, excluding Alzheimers.

Physical Disabilities Combined	83.4	72.0
Mental Health Combined	16.6	28.0

Note: Respondents indicated the three most frequent health problems of their patients. This table describes only the most frequent. Additional information showing all three responses is available.

TABLE 25: Participation in State or Local Organizations

Organization	OTRs %	COTAs %
Health Planning and Policy Groups	9.4	5.3
Business Groups	5.0	3.2
Education Groups (other than the PTA)	14.7	10.9
Health Related (other than state OT Assoc.)	18.0	11.9
Political, Gov't., Community Related	21.8	15.8

TABLE 26: Primary and Secondary Functions - OTRs

Function	Primary %	Secondary %
Administration	12.5	14.1
Consultation	6.5	33.1
Direct Patient/Client Service	72.3	16.6
Public Relations/Information	0.5	4.9
Research	0.5	1.8
Supervision	4.3	16.1
Classroom Teaching	2.5	2.3
Fieldwork Teaching	0.3	8.9
Other	0.5	2.2
Total	100.0	100.0

TABLE 27: Primary and Secondary Functions - COTAs

Function	Primary %	Secondary %
Administration	3.5	11.4
Consultation	1.5	24.8
Direct Patient/Client Service	88.5	12.3
Public Relations/Information	0.7	10.3
Research	0.2	1.1
Supervision	2.3	14.6
Classroom Teaching	2.3	5.9
Fieldwork Teaching	0.3	13.3
Other	1.0	6.1
Total	100.0	100.0

TABLE 28: Primary Age Range of Patients/Clients

Age Range	OTRs %	COTAs %
Less than 3 years	7.6	2.1
3 - 5 years	10.1	8.1
6 - 12 years	14.3	11.7
13 - 18 years	2.7	3.7
19 - 64 years	37.2	37.2
65 - 74 years	16.9	16.6
75 - 84 years	9.8	16.0
85 + years	1.3	4.6
Total	100.0	100.0
Pediatrics	34.7	25.5
Adult	37.2	37.2
Geriatrics	28.2	37.2
Total	99.9	99.9

TABLE 29: Self Employed and Private Practice

	OTRs				
	1973 %	1977 %	1982 %	1986 %	1990 %
Self-Employed*	6.0	12.3	15.0	19.5	26.4
Private Practice**	1.3	2.1	3.5	6.0	7.7
	COTAs				
Self-Employed*	3.4	8.0	4.0	6.1	11.3
Private Practice**	0.3	0.4	1.2	1.9	2.7

*Question asked was: Are you self-employed (that is, are you paid either on a contractural basis, or directly by your patient/client or his agent)?

**Chosen as a primary employment setting.

Annual Professional Income

*NOTE: The AOTA provides salary **for informational purposes only,** and disclaims any attempt to directly or indirectly suggest what salary schedule should be established for occupational therapist and/or occupational therapy assistants. The Association has to be very careful not to violate the antitrust laws in the collection or dissemination of salary and price information. The concerted use of salary and price information in a profession to restrain competition or fix prices is illegal.*

TABLE 30: Annual Professional Income by State

	OTRs +	COTAs +
Alabama	32,225*	22,675
Alaska	42,217	—
Arizona	36,912	20,591
Arkansas	34,561	—
California	39,810	25,238
Colorado	32,599	19,806
Connecticut	37,236	27,500
Delaware	36,828	—
Dist. of Col.	43,040	—
Florida	37,991	23,250
Georgia	36,892	24,238
Hawaii	33,173	24,038
Idaho	31,960	—
Illinois	35,133	20,136
Indiana	33,478	22,532
Iowa	30,930	16,618
Kansas	31,650	18,650
Kentucky	34,505	—
Louisiana	34,912	—
Maine	31,647	—
Maryland	37,637	24,154
Massachusetts	35,664	22,020
Michigan	34,838	21,435
Minnesota	30,800	18,441
Mississippi	38,742	—
Missouri	33,134	18,463
Montana	30,162	—
Nebraska	31,578	—
Nevada	42,408	—
New Hampshire	32,590	16,917
New Jersey	39,563	26,347
New Mexico	31,793	—
New York	38,797	23,365
North Carolina	35,052	22,333
North Dakota	30,884	16,818
Ohio	34,762	20,841
Oklahoma	33,745	23,844
Oregon	31,639	20,737
Pennsylvania	35,667	21,572
Puerto Rico	22,436	—
Rhode Island	37,957	—
South Carolina	34,701	—
South Dakota	32,118	17,700
Tennessee	35,093	21,036
Texas	35,999	21,348
Utah	32,837	—
Vermont	29,500	15,750
Virginia	35,578	22,000
Washington	31,869	18,323
West Virginia	36,036	23,500
Wisconsin	29,999	17,323
Wyoming	28,024	—

+ Full-time employed only

* Mean income

TABLE 31: Annual Professional Income by Employment Setting

Setting	OTRs +	COTAs +
College, 2 yr.	$38,438*	$24,464
College or University, 4 yr.	40,968	—
Community Mental Health Center	31,796	20,455
Day Care Program	30,670	18,828
Developmental Center	32,851	—
Early Intervention Program	30,476	—
Health Maintenance Organization (including PPO/IPA)	38,104	—
Home Health Agency	37,833	23,550
General Hospital - NICU	35,863	—
General Hospital - Psych Unit	34,129	21,786
General Hospital - Rehab Unit Only	33,159	20,700
General Hospital - All Other	35,161	21,713
Pediatric Hospital	33,962	21,792
Psychiatric Hospital	34,941	23,239
Outpatient Clinic, Freestanding	35,989	21,110
Physician's Office	37,117	—
Private Industry	40,658	29,045
Private Practice	44,306	23,438
Public Health Agency	36,824	22,550
Rehabilitation Hospital or Center	34,594	22,216
Research Facility	39,897	—
Residential Care Facility/Group Home/Independent Living Center	35,664	21,324
Retirement or Senior Center	39,136	19,700
School System	31,984	18,648
Sheltered Workshop	30,438	19,125
Skilled Nursing Home/ICF	37,055	21,256
Vocational or Prevocational Program	36,114	19,528
Voluntary Agency	31,429	19,700

+ Full-time employed only

* Mean income

TABLE 32: Annual Professional Income by Years of Experience

Years of Experience	OTRs +	COTAs +
0 - 1	$28,887*	$19,014
1 - 2	$30,333	$19,757
3 - 4	$32,734	$20,300
5 - 6	$34,382	$20,968
7 - 9	$36,350	$21,597
10 - 14	$38,532	$23,514
15 +	$39,005	$23,944
All Therapists	$35,470	$21,282

* Mean Income

+ Full-time employed only

Annual Professional Income

TABLES 33: Annual Professional Income (Employed Full-time)

Income	OTRs %	COTAs %
Up to $9,999	0.2	1.4
$10,000 - $11,999	0.1	2.7
$12,000 - $14,999	0.3	8.9
$15,000 - $17,999	0.5	18.4
$18,000 - $20,999	1.2	26.1
$21,000 - $23,999	4.3	18.8
$24,000 - $26,999	10.7	11.1
$27,000 - $29,999	16.4	5.2
$30,000 - $39,999	45.1	5.4
$40,000 - $49,999	14.3	1.4
$50,000 - $59,999	3.7	0.2
$60,000 - $69,999	1.4	0.2
$70,000 - $79,999	0.6	0.1
$80,000 +	1.2	0.2
Total	100.0	100.0
Mean	$35,470	$21,282
Median	35,000	19,500
Mode	35,000	19,500

TABLE 34: Annual Professional Income (Employed Part-time)

Income	OTRs %	COTAs %
Up to $9,999	15.4	37.3
$10,000 - $11,999	6.8	14.9
$12,000 - $14,999	12.6	15.7
$15,000 - $17,999	14.4	13.0
$18,000 - $20,999	11.3	6.5
$21,000 - $23,999	9.4	3.8
$24,000 - $26,999	7.9	3.5
$27,000 - $29,999	5.6	2.4
$30,000 - $39,999	11.9	1.4
$40,000 - $49,999	2.5	0.5
$50,000 - $59,999	1.1	0.5
$60,000 - $69,999	0.3	0.3
$70,000 - $79,999	0.3	0.3
$80,000 +	0.2	—
Total	100.0	100.0
Mean	$20,728	$14,346
Median	$19,500	$11,000
Mode	$9,000	$9,000

TABLE 35: Hourly Wage - Full-time Employed

Hourly Wage	OTRs	COTAs
Mean	$19.64	$12.98
Median	16.00	10.00
Mode	16.00	9.00

TABLE 36: Hourly Wage - Part-time Employed

Hourly Wage	OTRs	COTAs
Mean	$25.05	$12.39
Median	21.00	11.00
Mode	30.00	9.00

TABLES 37: Annual Professional Income by Primary Employment Function

Function	OTRs +	COTAs +
Administration	$43,884*	$28,386
Consultation	37,163	20,765
Direct Service/Treatment	33,345	21,040
Public Relations/Marketing	40,852	26,167
Research	41,030	—
Supervision	37,129	22,351
Classroom Teaching	37,374	22,161
Fieldwork Teaching	38,906	—
Other	35,272	24,364
Department Head	$37,796	$22,733
Non-department Head	32,446	21,005
Highest OT in Facility	$38,244	$22,833
Generalist Role	$34,742	$20,982
Specialist Role	35,620	21,791

+ Full-time only
*Mean income

TABLE 38: Annual Professional Income by Highest Educational Degree Level

Highest Educational Degree Level	OTRs +	COTAs +
Associate	$35,357*	$20,512
Baccalaureate	34,312	23,531
Masters	38,738	28,594
Doctorate	49,796	—
Other	34,694	22,144

+ Full-time employed only

*Mean Income

Reimbursement Sources

TABLE 39: Reimbursement Sources

Sources	OTRs %	COTAs %
Blue Cross/Blue Shield	6.3	6.4
Other Private Insurance	11.7	8.3
Medicare	23.6	26.9
Medicaid	9.6	13.5
Vocational Rehabilitation Agency (DVR/OVR)	0.8	1.1
Worker's Comp.	8.9	5.5
Other Federal Programs (Champus/OVR)	3.4	3.6
State/Local Programs	26.3	26.6
Patient/Client directly	4.3	4.3
Other	5.1	3.7
Total	100.0	100.0

Note: Each percent represents an average of all responses in the category. Only responses that totaled 100% included; does not include blank, unusable, "don't know" or "not applicable" responses.

Recommended Readings

American Occupational Therapy Association. (1979). *Occupational therapy product output reporting system and uniform terminology for reporting occupational therapy services* (1st ed.). Rockville, MD: Author.

American Occupational Therapy Association. (1989). *Guidelines for occupational therapy services in school systems* (2nd ed.). Rockville, MD: Author.

American Occupational Therapy Association. (1989). *Uniform terminology for occupational therapy and application of uniform terminology to practice* (2nd ed.). Rockville, MD: Author.

Bair, J., & Gray, M. (1992). *The occupational therapy manager* (2nd ed.). Rockville, MD: American Occupational Therapy Association.

Barros, A. (1990). The many faces of productivity measurement. *Medical Laboratory Observer, 22*(4), 17-18.

Brown, J., & Comola, J. (1988). *Improving productivity in health care.* Boca Raton, FL: CRC Press.

Cebulski, P., & Sojkowski, M. (1988). Clinical education and staff productivity. *Clinical Management in Physical Therapy, 8*(4), 26-29.

Chilton, H. (1990). Operational review: Beyond the numbers game. *Canadian Journal of Occupational Therapy, 57*(2), 95-101.

Cromwell, F., & Brollier, C. (Eds.). (1988). *The occupational therapy manager's survival handbook.* New York, NY: Haworth Press.

Dickerson, A. (1990). Evaluating productivity and profitability in occupational therapy contractual work. *American Journal of Occupational Therapy, 44*(2), 133-137.

Duncombe, L., & Howe, M. (1985). Group work in occupational therapy: A survey of practice. *American Journal of Occupational Therapy, 39*(3), 163-170.

Gilbert, J. (1990). *Productivity management.* Chicago: American Hospital Publishing Co.

Goldratt, E., & Cox, J. (1986). *The goal: A process of ongoing improvement.* (rev. ed.). Croton-on-Hudson, NY: North River Press.

Healthcare Information and Management Systems Society, American Society for Healthcare Human Resources Administration, and American Hospital Association. (1989). *Productivity and performance management in health care institutions.* Chicago, IL: American Hospital Publications.

Hertfelder, S., & Crispen, C. (Eds.). (1990). *Private practice: Strategies for success.* Rockville, MD: American Occupational Therapy Association.

Hopkins, H., & Smith, H. (Eds.). (1988). *Willard and Spackman's occupational therapy.* Philadelphia, PA: J. B. Lippincott Co.

Intagliata, S., & Hollander, R. (1987). The 3-hour therapy criterion: A challenge for rehabilitation facilities. *American Journal of Occupational Therapy, 41*(5), 297-304.

Jacobs, K., & Logigian, M. (1989). *Functions of a manager in occupational therapy.* Thorofare, NJ: Charles B. Slack, Inc.

Joe, B., Lawlor, M., Scott, T., & Thein, M. (1991). *Quality assurance in occupational therapy.* Rockville, MD: American Occupational Therapy Association.

Logigian, M. (1987). Productivity analysis. *American Journal of Occupational Therapy, 41*(5), 285-291.

Messer, T. (1986). *Simplicity in management of productivity and quality control.* Chicago: American Society for Healthcare Central Service Personnel of the American Hospital Association.

Miller, K. (1987). How rotation can help boost productivity. *Medical Laboratory Observer, 19*(1), pp. 52-56.

Punwar, A. (1988). *Occupational therapy: Principles and practice.* Baltimore, MD: Williams & Wilkins Co.

Riggar, T., Crimando, W., & Bordieri, J. (1990). Human resource needs: The staffing function in rehabilitation-Part I. *Journal of Rehabilitation Administration,* November, 99-104.

Schell, B., & Kieshauer, M. (1987). Beyond the job description: Managing for performance. *American Journal of Occupational Therapy, 41*(5), 305-309.

Scott, S., & Dennis, D. (Eds.) (1988). *Payment for occupational therapy services.* Rockville, MD: American Occupational Therapy Association.

Waters, C. (1987). *Splinting the burn patient.* Rockville, MD: American Occupational Therapy Association.

Wyrick, J., Ogden-Niemeyer, L., Ellexson, M., Jacobs, K., & Taylor, S. (1990). Occupational therapy work-hardening programs: A demographic study. *American Journal of Occupational Therapy, 45*(2), 109-112.